REIKI

Self Help Guide to Learn Reiki, Self-healing, and Improve Your Vibration Levels, by Learning Reiki Symbols and Tips for Reiki Psychic

(Raise Your Energy With Spiritual Growth)

Nina L. Mitchell

Published by Rob Miles

Nina L. Mitchell

All Rights Reserved

Reiki: Self Help Guide to Learn Reiki, Self-healing, and Improve Your Vibration Levels, by Learning Reiki Symbols and Tips for Reiki Psychic (Raise Your Energy With Spiritual Growth)

ISBN 978-1-989990-46-9

All rights reserved. No part of this guide may be reproduced in any form without permission in writing from the publisher except in the case of brief quotations embodied in critical articles or reviews.

Legal & Disclaimer

The information contained in this book is not designed to replace or take the place of any form of medicine or professional medical advice. The information in this book has been provided for educational and entertainment purposes only.

The information contained in this book has been compiled from sources deemed reliable, and it is accurate to the best of the Author's knowledge; however, the Author cannot guarantee its accuracy and validity and cannot be held liable for any errors or omissions. Changes are periodically made to this book. You must consult your doctor or get professional medical advice before using any of the suggested remedies, techniques, or information in this book.

Upon using the information contained in this book, you agree to hold harmless the Author from and against any damages, costs, and expenses, including any legal fees potentially resulting from the application of any of the information provided by this guide. This disclaimer applies to any damages or injury caused by the use and application, whether directly or indirectly, of any advice or information presented, whether for breach of contract, tort, negligence, personal injury, criminal intent, or under any other cause of action.

You agree to accept all risks of using the information presented inside this book. You need to consult a professional medical practitioner in order to ensure you are both able and healthy enough to participate in this program.

Table of Contents

INTRODUCTION 1

CHAPTER 1: WHAT IS REIKI? 4

CHAPTER 2: REIKI - UNIVERSAL LIFE FORCE ENERGY 8

CHAPTER 3: ABOUT REIKI 17

CHAPTER 4: INTRODUCING BREATHING TECHNIQUES 36

CHAPTER 5: HISTORY OF REIKI 42

CHAPTER 6: HOW TO STAY AT A HIGHER VIBRATION 62

CHAPTER 7: THE TALE OF REIKI 72

CHAPTER 8: WHAT DOES REIKI DO? 84

CHAPTER 9: THE BASICS OF CHAKRA HEALING IN 30 MINUTES OR LESS 98

CHAPTER 10: HEALING WITH REIKI 120

CHAPTER 11: HISTORY OF REIKI 139

CHAPTER 12: HOW TO BECOME A REIKI MASTER 149

CHAPTER 13: THE FIVE PHASES OF THE CHI CYCLE 154

CHAPTER 14: PERFORMING A TREATMENT 169

CONCLUSION 184

Introduction

In a world of faster connections, high-speed vehicles, instant communication, and a myriad of information at the tips of our fingers, we as human beings are often thrown off course. It is no longer strange for us to find ourselves trapped with problems of poverty, diminishing health, and the ever increasing cost of living. We are now used to taking pills for stress management, and stories about struggles- from the inner sanctum of the family, to the wars that are being fought for freedom and denied rights- no longer seem as new or frightening to us as they once were. We have become a race of chaos and imbalance. Though some of us are acutely aware that this is not how we must live, most of us have no idea that the universe, and our bodies, minds and spirits have already been given the solution to all of our problems.

Fixated as we are by the never ending tasks at work, the bills to pay, the children to care for, the career to develop and so on, we forget that life is more than just accomplishing everything we place in our calendars or planners. We forget that true living involves the development of a deep understanding of the self, others, and eventually, the cosmos. We forget that there is more to living than meets the eye, and that what most of us are doing is merely surviving. Many of us wake up every day, wondering how we have come to this, with problems looming over our head, worries and fears lurking behind our shoulders. Aren't you tired of that feeling- that feeling of helplessness, of being out-of-sync with the things that are truly important? Wouldn't you want to know how to raise yourself from the state of mere survival, to a state of utter peace, true understanding and transcendence to a higher, better version of yourself?

You already have the keys to the seemingly strange and locked door of limitless energy and profound meaning. Let this book teach you how to open all seven of your chakras, how to use them in your daily life, and how to recharge them with simple, proven techniques. Allow this book to take you on a life-changing adventure, and you will soon learn how to attain peace, how to block all the insecurities and fears, and how to live a fulfilling life. True happiness and the energy to engage in that state of happiness, is just a page's turn away from you. Read this book, open your charkas to the energy of the universe, and become one with your better, happier, and wiser self.

Thanks again for downloading this book, I hope you enjoy it!

Chapter 1: What Is Reiki?

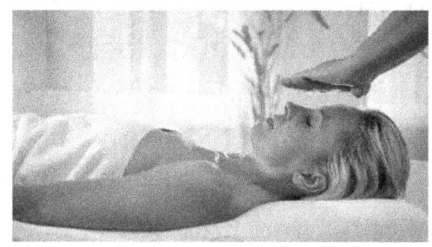

The word Reiki is a combination of 2 Japanese words. Rei refers to the higher power or God's wisdom and Ki refers to the life force energy which keeps us alive. Together, Reiki means "spiritually guided life force energy."

When you receive a Reiki treatment, it will feel like as if there is a magnificent, bright radiance or warmth flowing through and around your whole body. The sensations will be difficult to describe, but people who have experienced it say that one will always know once the energy has flowed through them. The good thing about Reiki is that it does not only treat the physical aspect but the emotional, spiritual and the psychological aspects as well. It provides a whole lot of beneficial effects like relaxation, peace of mind, security, stronger immune system and an improved overall well - being.

Reiki is actually very simple. It is extremely safe and is one of the most effective natural healing and self-improvement methods that you can use. People have seen its effectiveness, as it has been known to virtually help and treat every illness that there is. Coupled with therapeutic or conventional medical treatments, Reiki is a powerful tool that can be used to assist a person's recovery. There is no special ability that one needs to learn this simply Japanese technique. The only way to learn how to perform Reiki is by being taught by a Reiki master. The ability is passed on during a process called attunement. This is performed by the master during which the student is given the chance to tap into an infinite supply of life force energy. The energy is used to improve and treat conditions, as well as enhance the overall quality of life.

The use of Reiki does not depend on a person's intellectual capacity or spiritual development. Anyone who wants to learn Reiki can learn it. It has been taught to many people regardless of age, nationality and background.

Although Reiki is spiritual in nature, it is important not to treat it as a religion. It is based on no doctrine, which means there is nothing that you must learn or faithfully believe in order for you to learn and perform Reiki. Reiki does not make use of beliefs and will effectively work irrespective of your own views and beliefs on religion and regardless of whether you believe in it or not. Reiki may be used even if you simply believe in its intellectual concept, but since it still comes from God, a lot of people find that when they perform Reiki, they become more in touch with their religion. But even though you believe that you are more in touch with your religion when you perform Reiki, it is very important that you live and act your life in a way that promotes harmony with others.

One of the main purposes of Reiki is to help people realize that what's important is to heal their spirit so they can successfully improve themselves. The effects of Reiki will not last forever if you do not do your part. If you want the results to last, you need to play an active part in your healing and take responsibility. Aside from the energy itself, it is vital that you actively commit to improving yourself in order for Reiki to become an effective, complete system.

Chapter 2: Reiki - Universal Life Force Energy

What is Reiki?

How does Reiki Work?

Who can learn Reiki?

Benefits of Learning Reiki

What is Reiki?

Reiki is a Japanese word consisting of two characters "Rei" and "Ki".

Rei – Universal.

Ki - Life force energy.

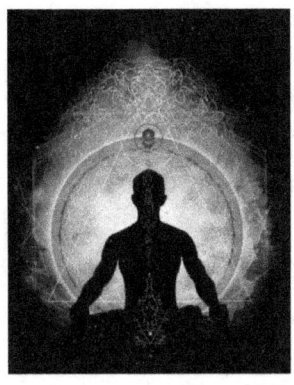

There is a non-physical omnipresent energy that gives life to every living organism in this world. The Japanese call this energy "**Ki**". It is also known as "**Prana**" in Asian cultures and "**Chi**" by the Chinese.

Ki energy can be developed or enhanced for the purpose of healing.. If a person's Ki energy is good and free flowing, he feels healthy and enthusiastic, he will be ready to face challenges of life and embrace the changes. If the Ki energy is low the person's attitude and thought forms will be negative, he finds it difficult to deal with life's challenges.

Ki energy is the very essence of the soul; this energy stays in and around our bodies from the moment we are conceived and it leaves the body when we die. This energy can be seen with the help of Kirlian photography.

Firstly Dr. Mikao Usui named this healing energy as "**Usui Reiki Ryoho**" which can be read as: **"Usui's teachings (dharma) to cure and heal one's True Self".** Later it got popular as Reiki.

How does Reiki work?

Basically, Reiki is a form of hands on healing; it clears emotional and physical blocks that lead to mental or physical illness. Reiki balances body, mind, heart and spirit in a gentle way through the healing light. Reiki can be used only for good purpose, all living things (plants and animals) respond to Reiki healing.

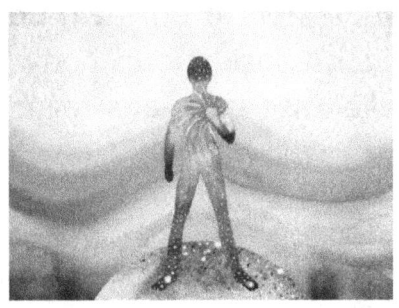

We all possess this natural gift and use it every day, although we don't realize that we are doing so. For an instance if we get hurt, automatically we place our hand on the sore spot and the pain will be relieved for a moment. Likewise, if your friend is hurt, a hug or tapping the shoulder will give some relief. This is how we unconsciously work with this energy to heal ourselves and our loved ones.

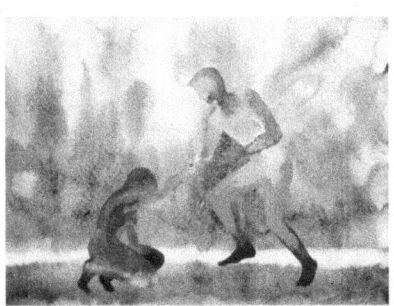

Reiki helps us to listen to our own bodies (what is going on inside our body and mind) and make wise decisions regarding health and well-being. Reiki is experiencing our "true self".

Reiki is a key to unlock our optimum capabilities. There are 7 main energy centers in the physical body that control the flow of the universal life force energy. These energy centers are called "the Chakras". Reiki opens up the chakras and enhances the energy flow. The best way to understand how Reiki works is to experience it.

Who can learn Reiki?

Learning Reiki doesn't depend on one's educational background, intelligence, or previous healing experiences. Anyone who is above the age of 9 irrespective of caste, creed, and sex can learn Reiki. The energy and information about Reiki is transferred from the master to a student through a process called Attunement.

Benefits of Learning Reiki

There are innumerable benefits of learning Reiki that can be used throughout life.

A few common benefits of learning Reiki are:

Develops compassion and gratitude

Increases patience

Relieves stress and anxiety

Builds good bonding in relationship

Improves health

Improves memory and concentration

Reduces tension and frustrations

Reiki is a natural pain reliever

Helps with pregnancy - bonding with baby and eases aches/pains

Aids better sleep

Helps with the grieving process

Clears fear, develops courage

Helps to follow your heart

Develops good communication skills

Increases energy levels

Increases self-love and confidence

Relaxes mind and body

Assists the body in cleansing toxins

Promotes strong intuition

Amplifies body's natural ability to heal itself

Helps to get good clarity, creativity and sense of purpose

Promotes emotional and spiritual growth

In order to get better results, one must purify one's thoughts and words and learn to meditate and let the **"true energy"** come out from within.

Reiki is not:

Mind controlling method

Escapism or doing nothing

Psychic surgery

Way to suppress emotions

Imagination

Pranic Healing

Massage technique

Superstitious ritual

'Uncaring', self-absorption

Secluded life

Shamanism

Psychotherapy

Chapter 3: About Reiki

The practice of Reiki has been around for a long time. It is the brainchild of Dr. Usui—a devoted Buddhist from Japan who mentored over two thousand people on the Reiki method right until his death. Reiki is "spiritually guided life force energy healing"—a kind of energy healing that works with the energy fields around the body. There are two root Japanese words Reiki stems from. "Rei" which means "Higher Power" and "Ki" which means "life force energy".

Why are we alive? It is because of a life force energy that flows through the compartment of our beings. We are full of life, vigor, and sound health if this energy is high in us. Otherwise, we stand the risk of illness. Just as in Energy medicine, this is the belief of Reiki. The technique originated in Japan and it is very useful for achieving relaxation and reducing stress levels. The Reiki energy is governed by spiritual principles and it is relayed through the laying of hands. The school of thought in energy medicine is that there can be energy stagnation in the body where there has been a physical injury or a case of possible emotional pain. In time, illness pops up when these energies are blocked. Energy medicine's belief and core ideology is primed at improving the flow of energy around the body. With it, the risk of illness can be drastically reduced while relaxation and speed healing are enabled.

The practice spread to the U.S. through Hawaii in the 1940s, and then to Europe in the 1980s. Reiki is the life force energy that flows through all living things. When we connect to the healing energy which is primarily resident in all human beings, we can tap energy needed for self-healing and general life. We can even help others. We have total health when our "ki" (energy) is free-flowing and solid. When the energy is weak or blocked it leads to symptoms of physical or emotional imbalances.

Reiki is available for everyone's use. From young to old, it is very safe and natural. According to studies and beneficiaries, it has been effective in combating all sorts of malady and sicknesses.

Quick Facts

Reiki involves energy transfer by hands-laying and it is growing in popularity despite lots of criticism.

Over a million adults in the US now find Reiki or a similar therapy useful and beneficiary to them health-wise according to a survey in 2007.[1]

Reiki is now becoming integrated into the hospital mainstream. It is now been suggested and offered professionally across Europe and the US.

Type "Reiki" into Google and you'll see close to a hundred thousand results. That is how popular it has become over the years.

There are studies all over, although not all over the place, that showed Reiki is effective for tackling pains among many other illnesses.

It Isn't a Religion

The Reiki ideology isn't something close to being attached to a religion because it isn't in any way. It needs you just the way you are. Its true source is from God. There are no set codes of belief you must adhere to before you can wield it. It has no dogma. Some people think a confident or self-assured mind means an added advantage to be able to use Reiki well, but that is not true. It needs nothing from you: skill, belief, confidence, values, etc.

Eventhough, it isn't a religion, Reiki does say you you should live your life with the consideration of some basic ethical principles. Harmony and peace with others are of great essence. And that is how you must live. There are certain ethical ideals, universal across cultures, which Mikao Usui—the Reiki founder—advised that everyone should live by to make the best of the wonderful technique.

A Bit of History

The body's energy system had to be understood. The revelation from it was what gave birth to Mikao Usui's version of Reiki. He wasn't the one that created it. He had rediscovered it. The initial practice and technique came to Usui in Japan after it had been passed from India to China and Tibet.

Everything about Reiki revolved around this great man called Mikao Usui. He had a sound education as his parents belonged to the wealthy class. He was committed straight at an early age to learning. That attitude helped him to master a lot early in life. He mastered Kiko also know as Chi-Kung. He also mastered how to use the sword effectively. He was so passionate and devoted that he would read just anything that gives a clue into how the human body works. That led him to be keenly interested in anything he could acquire from the field of medicine, psychology, and theology during his all-round and expensive education. One day, his life changed. It was a tricky question asked by one of his students while he was a teacher in a college. The question was: How did Jesus come about all the miracles said about him, especially the many sick people he healed? The question seemed strange.

The question had planted a seed and he was set on the path to find answers. It became for him a catalyst that pushed him into the deepest of committed research. He wasn't the one to shy away from that which seems mysterious. The students said that they were too young to believe, they needed proof. Before long, he left his post in the college and he went on a journey to find the answers. The knowledge of healing himself and others won't elude his searchlight. Such was his consummate passion.

Off to the holy mountains of Kori Yama. There, he fasted for good 21 days. He also meditated during those twenty-one days. Meditation would be needed as it would fast-track the receiving of the healing energy. It would raise him to an unprecedented state of heightened consciousness, he believed. By the morning of the 21st day, frustration had started building up, then just as he was about to leave in great disappointment, a great spiritual energy gushed down over him. Instantly he became consciously enlightened. Another gift he received was the ability to heal called "Reiki Ryoho". He was able to heal his hurting toe in no time by waving his hands over it.

Knowing that something profound had happened and that he was on the way to living a promising life, he returned to his monastery. A few days later he took his new knowledge to the slums of Kyoto that rims of beggars. For seven years he lived within them, treating their sickness and attending to all their avalanche of illnesses. As he was treating and restoring health to their beings, he was also training people the Reiki way as masters. Dr. Chujiro Hayashi, a retired naval officer, and a surgeon was one of the around-twenty prominent ones he passed on the torch of knowledge to. For ten months he had learned under the feet of Usui before his demise in March 1926. He would turn out to be the one that further popularized the Reiki system.

Dr. Hayashi was the next big thing that happened to the history of Reiki. After mastering Usui's system, the first thing he did was set up a Reiki clinic in Kyoto. The clinic attended to lots of people, both high class and low class and remained opened till 1940. It brought healing to many people and was seen by the public as something, not just beneficiary, but successful. His legacy involved the creation of a new Reiki style, yet still from the bowels of Usui—just some noteworthy additions. Hands positions were added so that all the aspect of the body will be covered. Several others became Reiki masters under his tutelage because of his improved system which made it teachable to many all at once. Just like he was to Usui, there was another named Hawayo Takata—a woman who took it up and spread it to the United States and the West at large.

Her entrance into the pages of Reiki history was somewhat unintentional. She was a beneficiary turned master. At a point in her life, she decided to visit Japan because of a prevailing issues she had with her health. She was getting knocked-off little by little and she thought a surgical operation would be the best option for her appendicitis and gallstones issues. Somehow, while in Japan, she thought she might not need a surgery again and decided to try and see if there was ever a way outside conventional medicine. The name on the lips of all she inquired from was a certain Dr. Hayashi. Scared and confused at first as to what alternative effort like Reiki could ever do for her debilitating health issues, she later gave in and reaped the result not too long there after. Her health was restored after several weeks of intensive Reiki sessions with Hayashi. Amazed, she asked to be taught how to transmit the energy to others so as to be of help. There was an agreement and from 1936 to 1938, she learned the first and second level of Reiki under Hayashi.

After she was done in Japan which was also one of her roots, the other been the US, she brought Reiki back home. Sooner, the West was suffused with this new technique of healing that is beneficial in ways altogether convincing. To step up her game, she lured Hayashi to come to visit her in Hawaii as she just opened a Reiki clinic. He agreed, her being one of his favorites out of the thirteen he attuned. There, he initiated her into the third degree of Reiki. Masters started learning at her feet in 1970 and she was able to add little tweaks also to the overall Reiki system. On the 11th of December 1980, she passed on. Her legacy to the generation after her was twenty-two Reiki masters—sound and effectively trained, and these ones became the torchbearers of the technique and directly responsible for its spread everywhere today.

What Is A Typical Reiki Session Like?

Reiki is nothing short of a major miracle as described by people. The powerful effect of a session lets the body get rid of a backlog of stress and tension. There is also the fourfold healing benefits of Reiki—physical, emotional, mental, spiritual. The feeling is like an exciting, splendid feel of a calming glow from the crown of your head to the sole of your feet. Around you, you feel like enmeshed in a pleasing halo of peace and perfect health.

The actual Reiki session is always an exhilarating experience. It is not restricted to a particular place or location. it can be held anywhere, so far as it's peaceful and filled with friendship. It starts off with the patient with full clothes on as he/she nestles on a table. A comfortable chair is also very common. Some soft, soul-lifting music could play underneath, but that depends solely on the patient's preference. The 60-90 minutes full session always provides a chance for the client to discuss problems he/she is experiencing and to discuss the expected results.

The actual session is very systemic and the practitioner begins it by using diverse kinds of hand shapes over the patient. The time spent per specific body area is always around 2 to 5 minutes in regard to the client's needs. In the occasion there are injuries or burns with the client, the practitioner's hands are maintained just above the spot in question. While the Reiki practitioner's hands are slightly over the patient's body, the actual energy transfer takes place in the client's system. The hands may develop a warm or tingling sensation and their positions are maintained until energy is sensed to have stopped flowing. The stop often times bring about a feeling in the hands of the practitioner and that is when the hands are removed from a spot and placed over another, and so on.

Reiki Techniques

There is only one Reiki but there can be some variation in the techniques employed. Some practitioners use crystals. Others use chakra healing wands. The thing about these aids is that practitioners find out that they can also enable healing and act as a reasonable negative energy protection choice for homes. However, in *Medical News Today*, Annie Harrington, Chair of the Reiki Federation of the United Kingdom (U.K) said:

"Reiki relies on no other instruments beyond the practitioner. We do not use crystals, powders or wands as a general rule. However, one of the benefits of Reiki healing is distance healing (where Reiki is sent over several miles) then, many practitioners will use crystals to assist with the energy vibrations."

Some of the techniques as used by a sound Reiki practitioner involve:

Extracting Harmful Energies

Beaming

Infusing

Centering

Smoothing and Raking the Aura

Clearing

Health Benefits

Experts versed in the knowledge and use of Reiki explain that modern scientific methods cannot be used to measure the life force energy that infiltrates the human body. It can only be felt by as those who stay tuned to it. Overall, Reiki is proven to aid the body's healing process in a very natural way. Apart from the peaceful feeling Reiki brings which is pronounced, it is helpful in taking the body to a seamless state of healthiness and well-being mentally, physically, emotionally, and spiritually. According to a study by the University of Minnesota, some of the common testimonials by those who have been exposed to the magic of Reiki sessions, revolved around:

great relaxed feelings

disappearing headaches after sessions

mental clarity

focused senses

heightened concentration levels

and feeling of calm sleeping.

"Intensely relaxing" was the word used for the profound benefits received by those who went through Reiki according to a study. Many other studies have proven that it aided a great deal in helping patients cope with difficulties. It also helped them relieve emotional stress and took their inclusive well-being on an upward trajectory. Perhaps because of its deeply-relaxing effect on the body is why cancer patients lay claim to a better feeling after receiving Reiki. The findings of Cancer Research U.K deduced that cancer patients feel better because the Reiki practitioner spends more time with them, and of course touches them. Some patients are overwhelmed by stress; others by fear of the invasive cancer therapy. The touch applied during Reiki helps a bunch.

Many cancer patients have found relief through Reiki's touch, same as those with chronic pains, infertility, and fatigue patterns, among many others. Many nervous system linked ailments such as

Alzheimer, Cohn's disease, autism, neuro-degenerative disorders are also helped by Reiki treatments.

Becoming a Reiki Practitioner

"Attunement" is the name attributed to a person's entrance into Reiki as a practitioner. It is a purely spiritual experience, so powerful, and it's the moment the student receives the entire package from the master. What is transferred through the experience, master to student, is the attunement energy and healing techniques. Entering Reiki's training is simple, free, and without any kind of retrains—personal or imposed. No prior training is needed; No set of dogmas and education is warranted, and no level of experience or personal profile is required.

What most students learn from the varieties of Reiki training available in the world today revolves around three things which are:

the ethics of practitioner-client situations

knowledge and understanding of the energies around the body

and working and mastering the healing energy.

There are set preparations that precede the Reiki attunement procedure. Fasting for 2-3 days is a crucial component as is meditation. Then there must be aspects that have to do with focusing on nature and releasing all negative emotions. Generally, there are three levels in Reiki and each has their significance. Only those that reach the Master level can teach others and can also heal from distance just like the way it works with prayers in Christianity.

Chapter 4: Introducing Breathing Techniques

I chose the specific quotation shown above for a reason. When you do yoga, you learn to breathe in rhythm with your movements. A lot of people put more concentration on the actual movements and not on the breathing techniques, but they go hand in hand and form part of the fluidity of yoga.

When you breathe correctly, you are able to use the inner energy better and that will push you further and that's why I feel that it is important that we pass a chapter on breathing techniques that will help you.

Posture

The first thing that you need to remember is that people who do yoga take up the lotus pose for a reason, but as a beginner, you don't have to take up the full lotus pose because it's complex and you may not be accustomed to bending your legs in such a manner. If it causes you discomfort, that's not the idea of the pose. The idea of the pose is simply this – to keep your back straight so that you are not interrupting the flow of energy through your body.

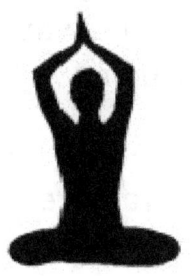

The true lotus pose means sitting with your back straight, bending your knees and tucking your feet in so that you form the shape shown on this small illustration. However, for newbies that's going to hurt. Instead, you need to get yourself a cushion to prop up your behind and then bend your legs at the knees and simply cross over your feet. This is easier and it helps you because your back is still straight. Instead of having your hands up in the air, you need to put your middle finger and your thumb together and place your hand, palm upward onto your knees. There's a good reason for this. One, it stops you from fidgeting and two – it actually gives you a sense of grounding which is important and helps you to concentrate on what you are doing.

When you have assumed this position, make sure that you are comfortable and that the clothing that you are wearing is not at all restrictive. Your concentration should be on your breathing, rather than on your waistband being too tight!

Breathing

Although you may argue that you know how to breathe since you are alive, breathing correctly is something else entirely. Concentrate totally and breathe in through the nose. What this does is take air into your upper abdomen. You should be able to sense the flow of the breathing and it's important that you concentrate on this and think of nothing else. Then hold the air inside you for a few moments and then let the air out of your mouth. You always use your nostrils for inhaling and can breathe out of your mouth.

Movement and breathing

This is a very important part of yoga. If you can imagine what it's like trying to singlehandedly push a piano from one side of a room to another, it's a bit like the effort that you put into exercises. It takes a lot of energy. No, try it another way and you will find that it eases the load. In yoga, you use breath in conjunction with movements because that extra energy that you get from breathing in the correct way helps the fluidity of your movements. As you make one movement, you inhale and as you change position, you exhale.

Exercise in breathing and movement

Hold your arms down by your sides. Inhale and move the arms up to above your head. You are doing this to get the breathing and the exercise working in conjunction with each other. Inhale — move hands stretched above your head — exhale, allow the hands to drop back to the side position. Don't expect to get this straight away. It takes practice, but when you want to do yoga effectively, you need to know what the inhale and exhale are what help you to gain more energy for your movements. Inhale — lift your arms up to the sky. Exhale, and relax them down to your sides.

It's a good idea to do this exercise regularly so that you get into the habit of practicing breathing and movement as much as possible because this helps your breathing and it also helps your movements to become more accented, more intentional.

Chapter 5: History Of Reiki

The Reiki strategy for recuperating was established on the disclosure and comprehension of the body's vitality framework. Reiki Practitioners endeavor to improve wellbeing and personal satisfaction by offering Reiki vitality and reestablishing harmony. Reiki is utilized in self-care, for consideration of one's family, and is offered in private practive and in emergency clinics and restorative settings as an aide and steady treatment to health and conventional medicinal consideration. The type of Reiki that numerous individuals practice today, Usui Reiki, has been being used for more than one hundred years.

The Founder of Reiki

The historical backdrop of Usui Reiki starts with its organizer, Dr. Mikao Usui. Now and again called the Usui Sensei, Dr. Mikao Usui was destined to a well off Buddhist family in 1865. Dr. Usui's family had the option to give their child balanced instruction for the time. As a tyke, Dr. Usui examined in a Buddhist religious community where he was shown hand to hand fighting, swordsmanship, and the Japanese type of Chi Kung, known as Kiko.

All through his training, Dr. Usui had an enthusiasm for drug, brain research and religious philosophy. It was this intrigue incited him to look for an approach to recuperate himself as well as other people utilizing the laying on of hands. It was his longing to discover a technique for recuperating that was unattached to a particular religion and religious conviction, so his framework would be available to everybody.

Dr. Usui voyaged a lot during his lifetime. He concentrated mending frameworks of various types and held various callings including journalist, secretary, teacher, community worker and watchman. At long last, he turned into a Buddhist cleric/priest and lived in a religious community.

Otherworldly Awakening and Development of Reiki

At some point during his long stretches of preparing in the religious community, Dr. Usui went to his very own preparation rediscovery course in a cavern on Mount Kurama. For 21 days, Dr. Usui fasted, contemplated and implored. Moreover, on the morning of the twenty-first day, Dr. Usui encountered an occasion that would change his life for eternity. He saw old Sanskrit images that helped him build up the arrangement of recuperating he had been attempting to design. Usui Reiki was conceived.

After his otherworldly arousing on Mount Kurama, Dr. Usui built up a facility for recuperating and educating in Kyoto. As the act of Usui Reiki was spreading, Dr. Usui ended up known for his recuperating practice.

Other commendable Development about Reiki

Hands-on mending has been logically demonstrated to be viable in quickening recuperating

A Reiki treatment bolsters the entire individual including body, feelings, brain, and soul-making numerous helpful impacts

On a physical level, Reiki enables reduction to torment, quickens the mending time of bones and wounds, loosens up muscles and decreases the tissue inclusion of consumes and wounds. It is conceivable to lessen the negative symptoms of medicines, for example, chemotherapy and radiation. Colds, cases of flu, honey bee stings, coronary illness - numerous physical conditions can be treated with Reiki.

On a psychological and passionate level, uneasiness is diminished, a feeling of prosperity expanded and another degree of unwinding felt. At this level of profound unwinding a rebalancing of energies happens and the common mending capacity of the body is improved

On a spiritual level, customers have expressed that they feel reawakened and restored after a full-body session

How is a Reiki treatment given?

A run of the mill Reiki treatment will see the customer lying full dressed on a back rub table. It is additionally conceivable to give a Reiki treatment to a customer sitting or standing. The professional places his of her hands on or close to the customer's body in a progression of hand positions from the head to the feet that are held for somewhere in the range of 2 to 10 mins, contingent upon how much time is required at each hand arrangement. The treatment will commonly last somewhere in the range of 45 mins to an hour and may incorporate input acquired by the expert during the treatment. A customer may profit to their professional for a fortnightly reason for some time or may locate that one session gives all the vital advantages. Reiki 2 experts are able to give separation mending meaning you could be anyplace on the planet and get recuperating from your professional.

What does a Reiki treatment feel like?

Everybody will have a somewhat extraordinary encounter anyway regularly individuals feel an a lot further feeling of unwinding. By and by I feel a stunning sparkling brilliance or vitality traveling through my body , here and there in floods and it will move through me and surrounding me. Others will see dreams, or feel like they are drifting over their body. Where the specialist feels blockages in a customer's vitality (and will invest time clearing that blockage) the customer may feel an underlying largeness however then a discharge and stream of vitality. It isn't unordinary for customers to encounter a passionate discharge as enthusiastic disturbance is brought to the surface and dischargeReiki is likewise a profound practice that develops genuine feelings of serenity, improves our wellbeing and essentialness, and advances mental prosperity. Every day self-Reiki medications are a solicitation to health: the establishment of thinking about ourselves and advancing parity and wellbeing on all levels. Reiki is the blessing that continues giving.

The word Reiki implies soul vitality or the vitality of the Universe, which is found in every single living thing, plants and creatures notwithstanding. As individuals, we are altogether brought into the world with Reiki; an attunement or reiju** is everything necessary to enable us to actuate or stir this capacity and recall all that we are able to do.

The training started with Mikao Usui in Japan back in the mid 1920s. Usui's involvement of illumination and deep rooted profound practice drove him to build up the recuperating technique we presently know as Reiki. He created Reiki as a profound practice to develop significant serenity in this way advancing wellbeing and prosperity. Usui Sensei skilled us with the Reiki statutes as devices for mental prosperity and profound development.

** Reiki is certainly not a substitute for medicinal, mental or other social insurance medications.

** A Reiki attunement or reiju is a delicate procedure or strengthening guided by the Reiki Master instructor to enable the understudy to open to, reconnect and line up with, the vitality of the universe and the mending limit that is as of now inside them.

The Reiki strategy for recuperating was established on the disclosure and comprehension of the body's vitality framework. Reiki Practitioners endeavor to improve wellbeing and personal satisfaction by offering Reiki vitality and reestablishing harmony. Reiki is utilized in self-care, for consideration of one's family, and is offered in private practive and in emergency clinics and therapeutic settings as an assistant and steady treatment to wellbeing and customary medicinal consideration. The type of Reiki that numerous individuals practice today, Usui Reiki, has been being used for more than one hundred years.

The historical backdrop of Usui Reiki starts with its originator, Dr. Mikao Usui. Once in a while called the Usui Sensei, Dr. Mikao Usui was destined to a well off Buddhist family in 1865. Dr. Usui's family had the option to give their child balanced instruction for the time. As a youngster, Dr. Usui contemplated in a Buddhist religious community where he was shown hand to hand fighting, swordsmanship, and the Japanese type of Chi Kung, known as Kiko.

All through his training, Dr. Usui had an enthusiasm for prescription, brain science and religious philosophy. It was this intrigue incited him to look for an approach to mend himself as well as other people utilizing the laying on of hands. It was his craving to discover a strategy for mending that was unattached to a particular religion and religious conviction, with the goal that his framework would be available to everybody.

Dr. Usui voyaged a lot during his lifetime. He concentrated mending frameworks of numerous kinds and held various callings, including columnist, secretary, preacher, community worker, and watchman. At long last, he turned into a Buddhist minister/priest and lived in a religious community.

At some point during his long stretches of preparing in the religious community, Dr. Usui went to his very own preparation rediscovery course in a cavern on Mount Kurama. For 21 days, Dr. Usui fasted, thought and supplicated. In the morning of the twenty-first day, Dr. Usui encountered an occasion that would change his life for eternity. He saw antiquated Sanskrit images that helped him build up the arrangement of mending he had been attempting to imagine. Usui Reiki was conceived.

After his profound arousing on Mount Kurama, Dr. Usui built up a facility for mending and instructing in Kyoto. As the act of Usui Reiki was spreading, Dr. Usui ended up known for his mending practice.

In the mid-1990s, there were disclosures of Usui's unique Reiki lessons. The commemoration of Usui was found by western instructors and a large number of Reiki's missing connections were revealed. Disclosures incorporated the revelation of a living Reiki custom in Japan, with extra strategies as instructed by the Reiki Gakkai (Reiki Learning Society). Some of Usui's notes and manuals were likewise shared, and this prompted more noteworthy disclosures which were later made all the more by and large accessible. Western

Reiki instructors increased new data seeing the framework as it had been educated in Japan and this was sorted out with setting up frameworks of Reiki in the West.

Usui's Students

On first September 1923, the devasting Kanto tremor struck Tokyo and encompassing regions. A large portion of the focal piece of Tokyo was leveled and completely pulverized by flame. More than 140,000 individuals were murdered. In one case, 40,000 individuals were burned when a flame tornado cleared over the open territory where they had looked for wellbeing. Tragically the quake struck in late morning, exactly when individuals' charcoal flame broils were set to prepare lunch. Three million homes were pulverized, leaving endless destitute. More than 50,000 individuals endured genuine wounds. The open water and sewage frameworks were obliterated, and it took a very long time for re-working to happen.

In light of this disaster, Usui and his understudies offered Reiki to incalculable unfortunate casualties. His facility turned out to be too little even to consider handling the crowds of patients, so in February 1924, he manufactured another center in Nakano, outside Tokyo. His notoriety spread rapidly all through Japan, and he started accepting solicitations from everywhere throughout the nation to come and show his recuperating techniques. Usui was granted a Kun San To from the Emperor, which is a high grant (much like a privileged doctorate), given to the individuals who had done respectable work. His acclaim before long spread all through the district also, numerous noticeable healers and doctors started mentioning lessons from him.

Usui rapidly turned out to be occupied as solicitations for instructing Reiki kept on developing. He voyaged broadly all through Japan, which was not a simple endeavor back then, to instruct and give Reiki attunements. This began to negatively affect his wellbeing and he started encountering smaller than expected strokes from pressure. On ninth March, 1926, while in Fukuyama, Usui kicked the bucket of a lethal stroke. He was 62 years of age.

It is said that Usui instructed Reiki to a little more than 2000 individuals and out of these understudies a few sources state he prepared 22 to educator level(Shinpiden). Huge numbers of these understudies started their very own centers and established Reiki schools and social orders. Not these educator level understudies are known outside of Japan.

By the 1940s, there were around 40 Reiki schools spread all over Japan. The vast majority of these schools showed the strategy for Reiki that Usui had created.

Dr. Chujiro Hayashi

The ancestry of most of Western Reiki experts springs from Chuijro Hayashi. Hayashi read with Mikao Usui for somewhere in the range of ten months preceding Usui's passing. He is accepted to have changed a portion of the strategies of Usui.

Chuijro Hayashi was conceived in 1879. At some point in 1925, Chuijro Hayashi met Usui. Chuijro had ascended to be an authority in the Imperial Navy and had prepared in Western and Chinese Medicine. In June of 1925, Hayashi got his instructor's preparation in Usui's framework. A few sources state that Chuijro Hayashi was a Methodist Christian, a reality affirmed one of his

Shoden/Okudent understudies, Mrs.Yamaguchi. Different sources state that he was a Soto Zen specialist who used the acts of Shinto.

Before his demise on tenth May 1940 Hayashi adjusted 13 understudies to the educator level, incorporating Hawayo Takata in 1938.

Mrs Takata - Usui Shiki Ryoh

Hawayo Kawamura (her original last name), was brought into the world 25th December 1900 in Hanamaula, Kauai, Hawaii. On the tenth March 1917 she wedded her significant other, Saichi Takata. They had two little girls, one named Alice Takata-Furumoto, who later had a little girl named Phyllis Furumoto.

It is because of Mrs. Takata that Reiki is outstanding and wide-spread throughout the world. Mrs. Takata officially brought Reiki to terrain America at the start of the

1970s and during a multi-year time frame, encouraged 22 Western understudies to the instructor level. Her style of Reiki created from what she was educated by Dr Hayashi.

It was following the demise of her significant other in 1930 and afterward her sister in 1935 that Hawayo Takata chose to go to Japan to visit her folks. Because of diligent work to help her family and sadness, Takata's wellbeing had started to endure. She was booked to have an activity in Japan to help settle her medical issues. Just before the activity, she heard the voice of her dead spouse, saying that the activity was a bit much and that there was another way. This provoked her to talk with her primary care physician about elective medicines, and he alluded her on to Hayashi's Reiki Clinic.]Hawayo Takata got day by day medications at this facility for a time of four months, and during this time her manifestations subsided.

This drove Hawayo Takata to take Reiki One preparing (Shoden) with Hayashi on tenth December 1935. She examined the principal level with him for barely one year. In 1937, Mrs. Takata got the subsequent level, Okuden. Soon after this, she came back to Hawaii. Half a month later, Hayashi visited Mrs. Takata with his little girl and remained until February 1938. During this time, Hayashi authoritatively made Mrs. Takata a Reiki educator.

Somewhere in the range of 1940 and 1970, Mrs. Takata ran a few Reiki centers and showed numerous classes in Hawaii. In 1973 she showed her five stars in the United States itself. In December of 1980 Mrs. Takata kicked the bucket. Much appreciation and affirmation is perceived for Mrs. Takata in empowering Reiki to spread all through the world. Without her, the arrangement of Reiki may have right up 'til the present time stayed obscure but to a chosen few in Japan.

Dr. Usui's Original Reiki Teachings

The more profound otherworldly practices and procedures of the Japanese conventions, notwithstanding, have stayed behind Japan's shut Reiki society. The first Reiki of Mikao Usui still thrives in Japan yet is impressively unique, practically speaking. Outside of Japan there are just three authorised educators of the pre-1922 framework — one of whom is an individual from The Reiki Guild.

Chapter 6: How To Stay At A Higher Vibration

By Justine Melton

Change is something that comes marching in when Reiki enters your life. The more you allow change to occur and are accepting of it the easier it is. Change comes best when you jump into the flow of the changing events and flow with it rather than swimming up the current fighting everything that is a change for your greatest good. One of the most common changes that comes with Reiki is the change in your vibrational level in the Universe. Usually after each Reiki attunement you will move up to a different vibration but it can also happen at any time.

When you manifest one of the most important steps is to allow yourself to feel as if you already have what it is you desire. This is actually you feeling the vibrational level of what it is that you are seeking. You have to send out the vibration to get the vibration.

Being at a higher vibrational level means that you are operating at a more positive level and are radiating that positivity and goodness to the universe as well. Good things flow to you more freely and it is harder to upset you. Some people term moving up a vibration as moving closer to enlightenment. One interesting thing that I have read over and over and have experienced first hand is that right before or after moving up a vibrational level you may feel like you are craving protein. It is believed that this occurs because your body needs the extra energy to make the jump to a new level. You may also notice that you suddenly need more sleep out of nowhere or that you are wanting to shed material possessions or things from different areas of your life that no longer suit you. If you happen to feel any of these know that it is quite common and that you are not alone. They are normal steps in a pretty incredible process.

Once you are at a new higher vibration you need to continue to live in a healthy manner in order to stay at the new higher state. Of course moderation in all things is important but overall it is important to maintain a healthy lifestyle to aide you in your quest up the vibrational ladder.

Ways to move to or stay at a higher vibration:

Reiki treatments (from others and/or daily self-reiki)

Saying no to anything that doesn't work for you

Letting what doesn't work in all areas of your life naturally fall away

Surround yourself in positivity

Eat a healthy diet full of fruits and vegetables and if you are a meat eater take note of how the animals were treated before and after they were killed. This can actually have quite an effect on the vibrational level of the meat you are eating. Also, chicken and fish have a higher vibrational level than red meat. A good rule is that if it has a hoof it is a lower vibration for you to consume.

Listen to up lifting music

Dance around your house... let loose

Do any healthy activities that bring a smile to your face

Exercise

Laugh

Let the sunlight hit your skin

Meditate

Keep a journal noting how different things AND people make you feel

If you need to say something say it. Do not keep feelings bottled in. If you are not comfortable telling someone something write it down on a piece of paper and wait a few days. The sooner you get it out the better.

Salt baths

Keep high vibrational stones/crystals around you such as tanzanite and quartz.

This is a general list for everyone but what I recommend most is to keep a journal for a week or 2 and write down any little thing that you notice that makes you feel happy or sad. If it does not make you happy it needs to go! This will have amazing effects on every area of your life and will aide Reiki in bringing the highest good into your life. Wishing you all love and light.

Strengthening Your Connection with Reiki

By Angie Webster

Sometimes practitioners worry that they

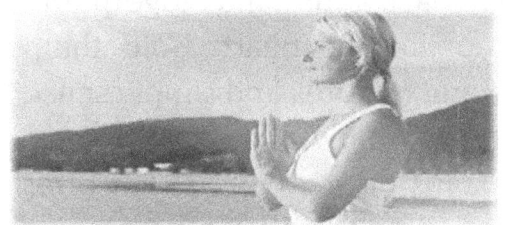

are not feeling very much energy flowing through their hands or their bodies. This is a question I receive quite a bit. I would like to address this by offering a few suggestions for strengthening the ways with which you can feel your connection with and your understanding of Reiki.

Reiki will flow through your body differently according to how it is needed in each situation and your perceptions will change from time to time as well, so that needs to be taken into account going in. Also know that there is no need to fear that Reiki is not flowing. However, I do believe that, with practice, we can become more aware of how Reiki flows through us and works with our individual systems.

Practice One: Place your hands together in prayer position at the heart. Hold them there for several minutes and simply sense how the energy flows in your hands. Notice the palms or any fingers that offer any sensation. Don't look for something specific. Your sensations are your own. Simply notice what is there. Breathe and notice and keep returning your attention to this area for at least 2-3 minutes, extending to five or so minutes a day. You could also try placing your hands at the third eye in prayer position for a portion of the practice and see what sensations you notice in your hands.

Practice Two: Briskly rub your hands together for a minute or so. Now hold them in front of your body, palms facing each other, about an inch apart. Gently and slowly push the palms towards each other but don't quite let them touch. Do you feel the gentle pushing sensation between your hands? That is the energy in your body. You may also sense a tingling or a heat in the center of your palms, or not. Either way is fine. Now try gently and slowly pulling the hands away from each other. Do you feel how it seems as if you are pulling taffy? The hands seem to be pulling toward each other. You are sensing the magnetic field of the body. These are ways the energy works in the body. Reiki is a part of that and the more you can tune into this, the more you will understand about how Reiki works in your body.

Practice Three: Do self Reiki every single day. Fit it in every way you can, using one hand while you do something else, if you need to. This is beneficial in the sense that your system is getting Reiki. However, if you are having difficulty sensing Reiki flow and you want to understand it better, you really need to take at least ten minutes or more a day to devote solely to self Reiki, so that you can notice how the energy moves through you, both in your hands and as it flows through your body. The subtle sensations may be very difficult to notice if you aren't tuned in with your awareness. Use it as a body meditation. If you feel you are too busy, all the more reason to slow down for yourself, your peace of mind and to honor your practice for ten minutes a day. All practices take some commitment and all skills take practice. It may help you to keep a notebook keeping track of what you noticed in your body, heart, head and hands each day. You may also choose to note a few simple things that you were dealing with in your life, physically, mentally or emotionally, so that you can begin to notice the changes that regular Reiki practice brings about.

Practice Four: Use Reiki on others often. This gives you a chance to notice the differences in the ways that Reiki flows with each person and each situation. Also, use Reiki in different life situations in everyday life. Use it on your food, in your bath, on your bed, your car before driving, everywhere you can think of! Practice, practice, practice!

Chapter 7: The Tale Of Reiki

Mrs Takata, a Reiki Master trained by Dr Havashi, (who was taught by and worked with Dr Usui) put the only history we have on tape. Not all facts have been confirmed but knowing what is truth and what is myth is not that important for the reiki practitioner. What matters the most is that Dr Ushui has left us with the simplest energy modality I know of. Once you have been attuned to reiki, all you need to do is think 'reiki on' to start the energy flowing and 'reiki off' to stop it. It's as simple as a light switch and I love the analogy. Other energy medicine can be as efficient but they usually imply learning about anatomy and physiology and directing the energy. The reiki therapist does not direct energy. He or she does not even need to know about the aura and the chakras. All is needed is to be a willing conduit for the energy to flow.

Mikao Usui Sensei, the founder of Reiki, was born on the 15th August 1864 in Miya Ma Cho, in the province of Gifu in the South of Japan. He was sent in his early age to a Buddhist Monastery. When he left, he obtained a doctorate in literature and travelled to China and various countries in Europe. There are many versions of the life of Dr Usui, not all can be verified. One of these versions states that although he was born onto a family of devoted Tendaï Buddhists, he only started to become interested in spiritual healing practices at the age of twenty seven, after going through a near death experience during a cholera epidemic. He then studies some sacred texts, the tantra, under the supervision of a master and monk of the Shingon esoteric tradition. He would have been the personal assistant of Pei Gotoushin, Minister of Interior and Prime

Minister of Tokyo. Some biographers pretend that he belonged for some time to spiritual healing school and that he learnt Rei Shi Jitsu, using energy to heal patients.

Another version says that he was a teacher in a Christian university and that one of his students asked him if he believed in the healing miracles performed by Jesus. When he said he did, the student asked him to demonstrate it. To understand the depth of Dr Ushui's predicament, one must know that in Japan, teachers are expected to be able to demonstrate everything they teach. Dr Ushui felt deeply challenged by the question and his lack of answer and felt he could not continue to teach as he had. He dedicated his life to finding an answer to this question. Some say he immediately resigned from his teaching position to start his quest on the healing methods of Jesus. This quest led him to travel the world. Whilst he could not find a proof of Jesus' miracles nor how

Jesus performed them in the scriptures, he came across some texts that in turn led him to study Buddhist scriptures. These scriptures intrigued him as they indicated that Buddha also had the power to perform miracles. So he started a journey to understand Buddhist scriptures and learn Sanskrit to decipher these sacred texts in the original language.

Back in Japan, at the Shin, Dr Usui asked a monk if the Buddhist Sutras gave accounts of Buddha healing. "Yes." He was told. He then asked if the Shin monks had mastered the art of healing the body. He was told, "We monks do not have time for the physical in reaching the spiritual growth. Spiritual healing is first." Dr Usui walked away into the jungle to visit other temples. Their stories were the same; none of the monastery monks could heal. His last stop was at the Zen temple. Here he heard again that the monks were very, very busy and had little time for the body healing — but they were sure that someday, during meditation, they would receive that great light and then they would know how to heal. Dr Usui decided to stay on and study all their secrets. He was then given permission to stay on at the Zen temple to do independent research. He spent the next three years studying the Sutras but without success.

Upon the advice of a Buddhist monk he studied with, Dr Ushui went on a twenty one day meditation on Mount Kurama, near Kyoto.

On the mountain he found an old pine tree near a stream. Here he piled up twenty-one rocks and watered them. He sat with his back to the tree with the rocks before him. After throwing one rock away, he began his first meditation. He expected a phenomenon of some sort but had no idea what it might be or when. He read scripture, chanted, meditated and drank water. He had no food with him. As the days and nights came and went the pile of stones dwindled. There was no phenomenon. Nothing. He used one rock per day.

On the twenty-first day, he woke before dawn and threw away the last stone. The morning black was near absolute – no moon and no stars. Dr Usui meditated, knowing it was to be the last time. On opening his eyes expecting to see nothing, there on the horizon, he glimpsed a flicker of light like a candle! He instinctively knew this was the phenomenon he had hoped for – and feared. Dr Usui braced himself, saying, "It is happening and I am not going to even shut my eyes. I shall open them as wide as I can and witness what happens to the light."

The light moved towards him seeming to accelerate as it approached. He was a bit frightened but decided to face whatever it was he had to face. With that he relaxed and, with eyes wide open, he saw the light strike in the centre of his forehead. When he came to his senses, he thought that he had died because at first he couldn't see and he felt nothing. The light was gone. He heard roosters in the distance and knew it would soon be dawn.

Dr Usui sat, dazed. Then, off to his right, coloured bubbles seemed to rise from the earth. Thousands of bubbles in rainbow colours danced before him then moved to his left. Dr Usui counted seven colours. And in those bubbles he saw the reiki symbols in gold letters. He was given the meaning for each of them and how to use them.

His retreat was over so he decided then to walk down the mountain. He was surprised to find no pain or hunger. "I feel my body is good. I'm going to stand up." He thought and he stood up. "My legs and feet are strong. I fast for twenty-one days, and still I feel I can walk back to Kyoto." His body felt well fed. "Well, this is a miracle – I'm not hungry and I feel very light." He dusted himself off, picked up his cane and straw hat. And then took the first steps of his twenty-five mile trek to Kyoto. Whilst he did so, he stubbed his toe quite badly, so that it bled and it throbbed. But when he held it, the pain disappeared instantaneously and the bleeding stopped. That was Dr Usui's second miracle that day. He then walked down the mountain and stopped by a food stall to have something to eat. He asked for a full breakfast. The seller who had seen many of these pilgrims come down the mountains knew it was dangerous for him to eat to much so he refused. But Dr Usui insisted so much that in the end he gave up. Dr Usui was able to eat a normal meal without any problems. That was the third miracle. The merchant's daughter had a tooth ache but because he couldn't afford a dentist, she was suffering in vain. Dr Usui offered to treat her, which she gratefully accepted. After only a few minutes of laying hands on her face, the pain vanished. That was the fourth miracle. Dr Usui then went back to the monastery to see the Abbot that had inspired him to go to Mount Kurama who was in a great deal of pain due to arthritis. Again, Dr Usui laid hands on him and the pain disappeared. Fifth miracle.

Dr Usui then went on trying to heal the poor in the slums of Kyoto for a period of seven years. His experience however, was that although he managed to heal the physical, nothing was done to change the mindset of the people he healed and most of them seemed to find their way back to the dispensary, having recreated their illnesses after only a couple of years. This led Dr Usui to write his principles for living to help the beggars take full responsibility for their lives. He realised that the patient's frame of mind about healing was paramount in the healing process. That the person must really want to get better and ask for healing for it to succeed. He found that when he offered his service free of charge, the recipient didn't actually value or appreciate what was offered, so he started asking for something in return.

Soon after, in April 1922, he opened a school of reiki and trained and initiated sixteen reiki masters. Mikao Usui was married and the father to two children. He died from a brain hemorrhagic on the 9th March 1926 at the age of sixty two, in the city of Foku Yama, near Hiroshima. He was respected and recognised by all, even by the Emperor of Japan who was deeply grateful to him. Mikao Usui was the president of an organisation called Usui Shiki Reiki Ryoho Gakkai, which still exists to date with the seventh successor to Dr Usui.

Reiki was brought to the West by Mrs Takata, who was the apprentice of Churijo Hayashi, an ex commander of the Japanese Marine Force. Churijo Hayashi was born in 1878. He was made a reiki master in 1925, aged forty seven, and was one of the last students of Dr Usui. He founded the clinic Shina No Machi in Tokyo. He died on 10th May 1941, aged sixty three. He initiated approximately seventeen reiki masters, one of them Hawayo Takata.

Hawayo Takata was born on 24th December 1900 in Hawaii. She suffered from a number of serious disorders including a tumour. Instead of going for surgery as was suggested to her, she decided to receive some healing. By a series of coincidences, she heard of Dr Hayashi's clinic in Tokyo and went there for several months of treatment. She came out free of her tumour. She stayed on and became Dr Hayashi's student. She was attuned to reiki I in the spring 1936 and went on to work as a healer in Hawaii. A year later she came back to do her second degree. She was made a reiki master in the winter 1938. She became Dr Hayashi's successor when he died. By the time she died in December 1980, aged eighty, she had trained twenty two masters, most of them westerners, including her grand daughter Phyllis Furumoto. Her students spread reiki to the West.

In addition to Chujiro Hayashi, Dr Usui had several other students, the closest of which were Jusaburo Ushida, Toshihiro Eguchi, Iichi Taketomi, Yoshiharu Watanabe and Keizo Ogawa. They each in turn has several students. The teaching of reiki remains very active in Japan, particularly through these generations of masters. Several western schools of reiki are inspired from these lineages and aim at perpetuating the original teachings of Reiki and to respect its authentic tradition.

Chapter 8: What Does Reiki Do?

People sometimes think that Reiki is a miraculous cure all – like a cosmic magic wand that will cure all ills. It is often marketed and sold as a healing tool that will take away all your worries, concerns and illness.

This is NOT what Reiki does.

"Reiki doesn't remove, it uncovers, it clears away the confusion to help us recognise and identify the underlying causes that need our attention in order that we can begin to help and heal ourselves. The belief that Reiki is a miracle cure is far more palatable to most people, and easier than the reality of helping you get your shit together." **- Phillip Hawkins – "Reiki hold my beer I've got this!"**

This quote sums up exactly what Reiki does. It shines the light into the dark corners and illuminates what needs to be addressed. Healing is a matter of deep personal introspection, being brave enough to look into the shadows and face what is there. It helps you bring to the surface all the things that are holding you back.

Usui himself knew that in order for healing to take place, we must take an active role and make changes in our own lives. He called Reiki "his system" – the word Reiki was given to this system later, along with the hand positions, symbols and other hoops we now all tend to jump through.

Usui recognised that we are all connected to this life force within us and around us and that true healing comes from within. Reiki is a system of personal and spiritual development – the healing of others is simply a side effect of the work we do on ourselves.

It's funny how from a physical perspective we will certainly change things if we hurt ourselves. For example if you burn yourself you learn not to put your hand in the fire again or if you cut yourself you know not to pick the scab and allow it to heal.

From an emotional or spiritual perspective though we tend to repeat patterns and then wonder why we are still hurting. Still having negative thoughts and repeating a cycle of behaviour. Reiki helps you see what changes need made and then it is up to you to decide to make those changes.

So how does Reiki work?

Life force energy – also known as chi, ki, prana, etc., flows through our bodies in energy pathways called meridians. As well as flowing around the body it also flows in and around our aura – the field of energy that surrounds us.

This energy field responds to everything we say, think and feel and when we are surrounded by negativity or if we are thinking negative thoughts then blocks and imbalances can occur in this energy field.

We are unconsciously absorbing everything around us all the time so Reiki works to help clear these blocks and imbalances.

If these imbalances and blocks are not cleared they gradually become more dense over time and eventually lead to physical illness or disease in the body. Because Reiki energy vibrates at such a high level it easily breaks up and clears these blocks and imbalances.

It charges the energy field with positivity and love – it balances out the chakras (the body's energy centres) and allows life force to flow cleanly around the entire system.

It strengthens and accelerates the body's own natural healing abilities. It also gradually begins to open the mind, heart and spirit to accept and understand the deeper levels of healing needed.

It is an intelligent energy that finds its way to where it is needed most so each time you have Reiki you receive exactly what you need.

Do you need to be spiritual for it to work?

Not at all – Reiki will work whether you believe in it or not. It is better if you can approach it with an open mind and allow it in but Reiki will work nonetheless.

You do not have to have any specific religious or spiritual belief – it is not a religion or cult. If you do have a belief in a higher power then you can incorporate Reiki into that belief system. I have many Christian students who see Reiki as coming from God or Jesus. I have Pagan students who see Reiki as part of nature. I have Muslim students who see Reiki as coming from Allah. Whatever your belief system, Reiki can fit in. It is simply the timeless and profound healing energy of the Universe.

The principles are simply there to help you work on your own healing. Please remember that 'Reiki' is the system that Usui re-discovered. The energy it is based on, is as ancient and timeless as the Universe itself.

So what are the principles & what is the Reiki philosophy?

Usui formulated the following principles while developing the Reiki system as we know it: –

Let's take a look at these principles in a little more detail – I will go into each one in a deeper way over the next few chapters so that you get a full understanding of them but for now I will simply touch on each one.

"Just for today" – this is such an important principle.

Quite often when you try to change your mindset or give up a bad habit you get overwhelmed by the enormity of the situation and the fact that "forever" is a very long time.

By incorporating the "just for today" approach you can break down your changes into manageable chunks. For example it is easier to say that just for today I won't eat that chocolate cake rather than saying I will never eat chocolate cake again.

The other part of the "just for today" concept is that you learn to live in the moment.

Today is a collection of moments. This concept teaches us to fully live in the moment each day.

Mindfulness is a very powerful thing and can encourage greater happiness and well-being.

I want you to take a moment now to check in with your body –

- How are you sitting or standing?

- Is your head up straight or tilted to the left or right?

- Are your shoulders hunched or relaxed?

- What is your mouth doing – is it smiling or are your teeth clenched?

- Are you warm or cold?

- How are you breathing – deeply or in a shallow manner?

This simple exercise puts you in the moment and this is one of the keys to the Reiki philosophy. Just for today – in other words, live in the now.

Let's try another exercise –

I want you to simply breathe in and out and on the in breath say the word "Here" and on the out breath say the word "Now" - take a moment to do that now.

How do you feel now?

I bet you are more relaxed than before? This is a wonderful practice to do each day and it really puts you in the present moment!

So let's move on – Principle 1 - Do not anger.

You can recover the balance of mind and emotion with Reiki. Anger just hurts yourself and others. It is a negative emotion which has no place in Reiki.

Using the "just for today" concept you can learn to become mindful and recognise when anger is bubbling up. Just by stopping and taking a moment to recognise it you can often remove yourself from the situation or choose to react differently.

Anger is a loss of control. When you work with Reiki energy and meditation you can recover this loss of control and transmute the anger into a more positive response.

Quite simply being angry is a conscious choice – often just a habitual reaction to a set of circumstances – so with practice, we can choose not to be angry.

Principle 2 - Do not worry.

Learning Reiki and using it daily is the step for learning to fully trust the universe.

Do not have any unnecessary worries or fears. Do your best today and let the universe take care of the rest – keeping your mind peaceful. It is the key to being able to fully trust that you release all fear.

Worry comes from fear and from having a "what if" mentality. Practising mindfulness and using these principles you can choose not to worry and choose to stay in the here and now.

Principle 3 - Be Grateful.

As you use Reiki and become Reiki you naturally become more thankful and grateful for the gift that is Reiki. You begin to realise that we are all connected and that the universe is inherently abundant.

Being grateful opens you up to receiving more lovely experiences from the universe as you raise your energy frequency to be thankful for what you have rather than complaining about what you don't.

Principle 4 - Work hard on yourself (sometimes translated as do your work honestly).

This just means that you will work hard – not that you normally don't do honest work! It promotes working hard for what you want – it doesn't mean you have to be unhappy in your work rather it promotes that you work at something you love in order that you can happily do it and be honest with yourself daily.

You can use Reiki in your daily life and work. A lazy mind is bad for you. People grow through work and learn through everyday life. It means to be true to yourself and to work hard on yourself and your spiritual development.

Reiki is a disciplined practice which becomes a lifetime journey of learning and development if you let it.

Principle 5 - Be kind to others.

A sense of oneness can be developed naturally through Reiki healing. Reiki is a practice of love. A healthy society can only be established through the co-operation of a large number of people.

In the universal dimension there is no distinction between self and others, only the existence of the same soul. Be kind to others is therefore synonymous to be kind to yourself.

Just think the more people that learn Reiki and become Reiki, the more people will live by the principles above and how much better will that make our world?

Usui's memorial stone reads: –

I think that is just beautiful, and something to aspire to.

Chapter 9: The Basics Of Chakra Healing In 30 Minutes Or Less

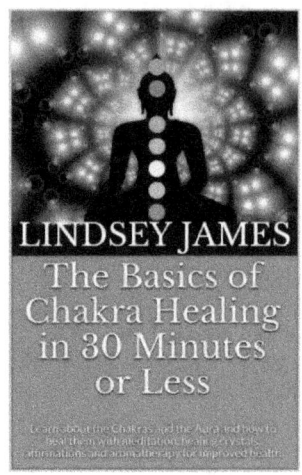

Learn about the Chakras and the Aura and how to heal them with meditation, healing crystals, affirmations and aromatherapy for improved health and wellbeing

INTRODUCTION TO CHAKRA HEALING

This book is an introduction to Chakra healing and explains some techniques for healing Chakras with meditation, healing crystals, affirmations and aromatherapy.

When you have finished reading this book, which typically takes 30 minutes or less for most people, you will have a basic understanding of Chakras and the Aura and be ready to start healing your Chakras for improved health and wellbeing.

CHAKRAS AND THE AURA

We all possess an energy field, known as an aura, which both fills and surrounds our bodies. This is connected to the universal energy field by spinning wheels of energy known as Chakras.

Between the base of your spine and top of your head there are seven major Chakras. A blockage in any of your Chakras can cause you to suffer from physical or psychological ailments.

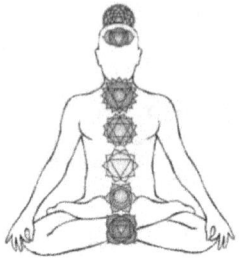

7. Crown Chakra
6. Third eye Chakra
5. Throat Chakra
4. Heart Chakra
3. Solar plexus Chakra
2. Navel Chakra
1. Root Chakra

Physical illnesses are often the result of psychological challenges. Our mental, emotional and physical health must all be in perfect balance in order for our bodies to function at their best. Our Chakras work to preserve that balance.

Knowing how to maintain balance within your Chakras and how you are affected by them is vital. If the Chakras are in proper alignment many ailments can be overcome or effectively managed.

The first Chakra is the root Chakra which enables you to feel safe, grounded and responsible. If it becomes imbalanced, you might feel insecure or anxious. On a physical level, your legs, sexual organs or hips may be affected. Symptoms include muscle cramps, pain in the legs and feet, decreased libido, and lower back pain.

The second Chakra is the navel Chakra which governs confidence and the ability to engage in relationships and relate to other people. If your navel Chakra is out of balance you may become fearful, apathetic, and distrusting of others. You may also struggle to form long term relationships, become sexually absorbed or manipulative.

Physically the navel Chakra is responsible for large intestines, sex organs, bladder and kidneys. Symptoms of Chakra imbalance include constant urination, lower back pain, impotence, cysts and infertility.

The third Chakra is the solar plexus Chakra. This Chakra works to maintain health in your gallbladder, pancreas, small intestine and liver. It also controls impulse, anger, passions and ego.

Rash or irate behavior, addiction and emotional instability are signs that your solar plexus Chakra is blocked or out of balance. Physical symptoms include indigestion, intestinal problems, liver disorders, food allergies and diabetes.

The fourth Chakra is the heart Chakra which both physically and metaphorically is responsible for your heart as well as your lungs, upper back and circulation. It affects heart function as well as any love in your life. Psychologically the fourth Chakra connects your body, spirit and mind.

Inadequate coping skills, schizophrenia, phobias, unfaithfulness and neuroses are signs that the fourth Chakra is not balanced.. Other symptoms include heart problems ,asthma, insomnia, back pain, pain in the upper arm, sore shoulders, some cancers and high blood pressure.

The fifth Chakra is the throat Chakra, responsible for your mouth, ears, throat and thyroid. On a psychological level you may become unable to express emotions, anger in particular. Other mental symptoms include decreased confidence, depression, confusion, insecurity and shyness. Bodily you might become inflicted with ear infections, gum disease, sore throat, hyperthyroidism and other ailments.

The sixth Chakra is the third eye Chakra which controls intuition or your ability to see beyond the obvious. It is responsible for your face, brain and eyes. Mental symptoms of a blocked or out of balance sixth Chakra include negativity towards others and selfishness. Physical symptoms include migraines, jaw pain, blurred vision, glaucoma and cancer.

The seventh Chakra is the Crown Chakra. This Chakra provides insight and wisdom.

It is because of the seventh Chakra that you are aware of the world and your place in it. If your crown Chakra becomes imbalanced you may feel neurotic, fearful, frustrated, or even psychotic. Your general well-being can be affected and you might feel extremely sad or lost and depressed.

Many common ailments are the result of imbalanced Chakras. If you are suffering with emotional problems or physical illness or you feel mentally or physically burnt out, healing your Chakras could bring positive changes in your life.

CHAKRA HEALING WITH MEDITATION

Meditation can be done informally while sitting comfortably in a chair. It is best to meditate somewhere quiet so you can concentrate without interruption. Successful mediation requires you to completely relax and clear all worries and distractions from your mind.

To get ready for meditation, sit in a comfortable position, deliberately relax your muscles, let your breathing slip into a constant rhythm and clear all thoughts from your mind.

At first you might have difficulty keeping your mind clear. As you are not physically engaged in any activity, your mind might wander. Should this happen, make a deliberate effort to clear your thoughts and continue your meditation.

Using chants and symbolic gestures can help to stop your mind from wandering as you will get into a rhythm of breathing and vocalizing the chant. Chants and gestures, which are known as mudras, are explained for each of the Chakras on the following pages.

Relax, settle your breathing and form the mudra for the Chakra that you want to focus on. Visualize the location and color of the Chakra and vocalize the chant each time you breath out.

Meditate as long as you can comfortably do so. If keeping a clear mind becomes arduous, or you begin to feel uncomfortable it is time to stop.

It is not necessary to meditate for any specified period of time. In the beginning, you might find it challenging to meditate longer than a few minutes. However, with practice you should be able to meditate for longer periods.

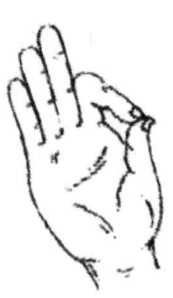

The mudra and chant for each Chakra are explained below. When meditating, visualize the location and color of the Chakra and repeat the chant several times.

FIRST OR ROOT CHAKRA

Hands resting on knees, open with the tips of the index finger and thumb touching.

Chant: Lam, pronounced *l-a-a-a-a-a-m*

SECOND OR NAVEL CHAKRA

Hands in lap, palms facing upwards with the right palm resting on left, tips of thumbs touching.

Chant: Vam, pronounced *v-a-a-a-a-a-m*

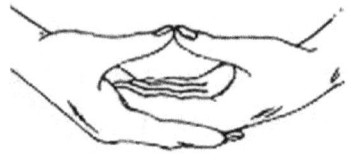

THIRD OR SOLAR PLEXUS CHAKRA

Hands together facing away from the body between heart and stomach with one thumb on top of the other.

<u>Chant:</u> Ram, pronounced *r-a-a-a-a-m*

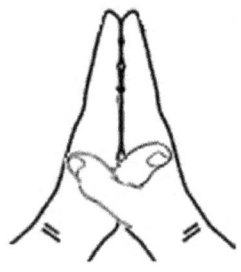

FOURTH OR HEART CHAKRA

Right hand in centre of chest and left hand resting on knee, both with tips of the index finger and thumb touching.

Chant: Yam, pronounced *y-a-a-a-a-m*

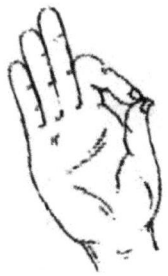

FIFTH OR THROAT CHAKRA

Hands in front of stomach with fingers interlaced and tips of thumbs touching.

Chant: Ham, pronounced *h-a-a-a-a-m*

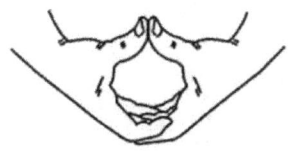

SIXTH OR THIRD EYE CHAKRA

Hands together with middle fingers raised and tips touching at level of chest, all other fingers touching at the knuckles.

Chant: Aum, pronounced *a-a-a-u-u-u-m*

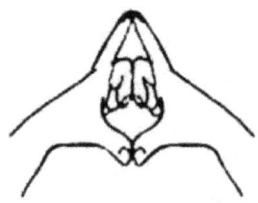

SEVENTH OR CROWN CHAKRA

Hands interlaced in front of stomach with little fingers pointing upwards.

Chant: Ang, pronounced *a-a-a-a-a-n-g*

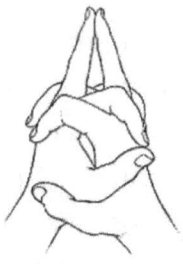

CHAKRA HEALING WITH CRYSTALS

Crystal healing, also known as crystal therapy, is a type of vibrational medicine that uses life force energies controlled by the Chakras.

Crystals are believed to have the ability to align body vibrations and release the Chakras life force energies in order to unblock them and restore their balance.

If you would like to learn more about utilizing crystals for healing, there are several books on the subject. However, I will go over some general methods of using crystals to balance the Chakras.

Crystals must be cleansed before use in order to remove energies absorbed during handling. Next they must be dedicated and energized for your particular needs. Additionally, crystals must be energized and cleansed before and after every use.

You can simultaneously energize and cleanse most crystals by setting them in a bowl under running water for 10 minutes.

Dedicating, or programming, the crystal for its new purpose is simple. Just find a quiet place where you will not be interrupted, hold the crystal before you, then clearly think or state your purpose while concentrating on the crystal. It can be as simple as "I dedicate this crystal for healing" or something more specific.

There are many methods for using crystals to balance the Chakras. Some people carry crystal tumble stones in their pockets or wear jewelry that incorporates the crystal.

Others prefer to massage in the area of the Chakra with the crystal.

You may also hold them in your hand, against the area of the Chakra, or close to it, while you mediate. Another method is to place the crystals on your body while lying down, though you might need a friend's help to do this.

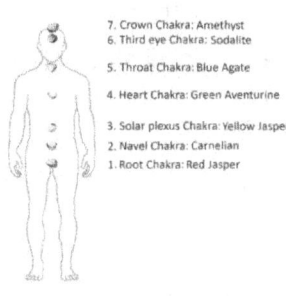

7. Crown Chakra: Amethyst
6. Third eye Chakra: Sodalite
5. Throat Chakra: Blue Agate
4. Heart Chakra: Green Aventurine
3. Solar plexus Chakra: Yellow Jasper
2. Navel Chakra: Carnelian
1. Root Chakra: Red Jasper

Crystal healing practitioners use a technique referred to as the laying on of stones to bring balance to the Chakras. Energies in the stones help reset the vibration and energy flow of the Chakras when placed on them and other parts of the body.

A layout that is commonly used is to place a single crystal on the body at the location of each Chakra. Either clear quartz or a crystal of the color associated with each Chakra are used. A typical selection of crystals for Chakra healing is shown in the following illustration.

A selection of suitable crystals for placement on each Chakra is shown in the following list.

First or root Chakra: Garnet , Red Jasper, Ruby

Second or navel Chakra: Carnelian, Fire Opal, Orange Calcite

Third or solar plexus Chakra: Citrine, Honey Calcite, Yellow Jasper

Fourth or heart Chakra: Emerald, Green Aventurine, Malachite

Fifth or throat Chakra: Aquamarine, Blue Agate, Turquoise

Sixth or third eye Chakra: Lapis Lazuli, Sodalite, Sapphire

Seventh or crown Chakra: Amethyst, Clear Quartz

CHAKRA HEALING WITH AFFIRMATIONS

To heal your Chakras with meditation, find a quiet place where you can lie down or sit. It is not necessary to say the affirmations out loud, but you can if you wish.

Here are some affirmations that you can use for each of your Chakras. As you speak or meditate on each one, focus on the location of each Chakra and think of its color.

First or root Chakra: I am a divine being of light, and I am peaceful, protected and secure.

Second or navel Chakra: I am radiant, beautiful and strong and enjoy a healthy and passionate life.

Third or solar plexus Chakra: I am positively empowered and successful in all my ventures.

Fourth or heart Chakra: Love is the answer to everything in life, and I give and receive love effortlessly and unconditionally.

Fifth or throat Chakra: My thoughts are positive, and I always express myself truthfully and clearly.

Sixth or third eye Chakra: I am tuned into the divine universal wisdom and always understand the true meaning of life situations.

Seventh or crown Chakra: I am complete and one with the divine energy.

CHAKRA HEALING WITH AROMATHERAPY

Some people use aromatherapy to heal the Chakras. Techniques include massaging the location of the Chakra with essential oils diluted with a carrier oil, adding essential oils to a bath and diffusing essential oils for inhalation.

Essential oils believed to be beneficial in healing the individual Chakras are shown in the list below.

First or root Chakra: Cedarwood, patchuli, sandalwood, vetiver

Second or navel Chakra: Jasmine, juniper, rose, rosemary, sandalwood

Third or solar plexus Chakra: Bergamot, juniper, lavender, rosemary, vetiver

Fourth or heart Chakra: Cedarwood, rose, sandalwood

Fifth or throat Chakra: Lavender, patchuli

Sixth or third eye Chakra: Geranium, lavender, rosemary, spearmint

Seventh or crown Chakra: Frankincense, jasmin

For massage, make a blend of up to 10 drops of essential oil per ounce of a suitable carrier oil such as grapeseed oil and gently massage the location of the Chakra.

For bath oil, Blend 10 drops pf lavender oil with 1 ounce of carrier oil. This will make enough for four baths and should be stored in a glass bottle.

Mix a quarter of the mixture into a hot bath just before you get in.

If you want to diffuse essential oils for inhalation, follow the instructions for your diffuser. If you do not have a diffuser, add a few drops of essential oil to a cup of boiling water or place a few drops of essential oil on a paper tissue.

Essential oils can be harmful if used improperly so always observe safety precautions when using or handling.

The National Association for Holistic Aromatherapy provides comprehensive safety advice on their website at:

Chapter 10: Healing With Reiki

As mentioned in the previous chapter, Reiki healing can only be done for the greater good and a practitioner should not really abuse or misuse it. Reiki energy can be used to heal any part of a person, including the body, the mind, and even the soul. It can work in all chakras and in all emotions. It can work on your spirit or on your karma. Reiki energy can go into your past, your present, or your future. Reiki energy can heal any part of your being, including all your relationships with other people and any other aspect of your life. You just need to have the faith that it can heal exactly what needs to be healed.

Reiki healing will always use its powers for your greatest good, even if you do not really know what that particular thing is yet. If the Reiki healing that you perform on yourself or on another person is not really required at that particular time, be assured that it will not go to waste because the Reiki energy will be sent to heal at a later time – when it is the right time.

Self-Healing

When you have a real intention to become healed and be happy and when you can be fully committed to change yourself for the better, you have already begun your journey toward self-healing. When you have real faith and trust in the divine guidance that can heal you, you will begin to feel your load being lifted from your own shoulders and you will sense that you are traveling toward the right direction.

During the healing process, you can have varying emotions that can range from intense love and joy to moments of great pain and grief. As you may already know, change always happen in your life, in everyone's life. Some changes are small and seem insignificant whereas others are a lot bigger and seem more frightening. But you must know that all the changes that you will experience through life will lead you to that special place where there will be more happiness than you have ever experienced in your life.

When you are able to engage the truth and find out that you actually do not have anything to fear, you will be able to take off a heavy suit of armor you have always worn to protect yourself from all of the things you fear. This heavy suit of armor has actually become a barrier that keeps you from successfully moving toward a happy and fulfilled life because it cannot really protect you when what you really fear is not from the outside but from deep inside you. When you are able to finally take off your suit of armor, you will be able to breathe more effortlessly, view things more clearly, experience the pleasurable feelings of the sun, the rain, and the wind, and you will be finally set free from the imprisonment you have imposed upon yourself.

You may have experienced substantial trauma and distress at some point in your life. The wounds from those hurtful life experiences is one of the things that you need to heal in yourself. If you still feel pain from being separated from a loved one because of death or other reasons that had an intense impact in your life, you need to heal the pain so you can move on from that traumatic experience toward a happier and more fulfilled life. Each one of us has our own coping mechanisms for the various traumas we experience in life. But your coping mechanisms may involve closing off a part of yourself hidden deep inside your being and you allow your subconscious to protect you from any more harm and pain by all means.

But even when you have a sturdy protection in place, it does not mean that the pain and wounds that you have buried deep inside that protection have already been healed. Your coping mechanism or your "heavy suit of armor" can keep a particular part of you clogged up and closed off, which can be manifested as insecurity, a reluctance to give and receive love, or the incapability to feel certain emotions.

When you have learned how to achieve attunement with Reiki energy, you will be able to easily bestow upon yourself Reiki healing. You will simply have to use specific hand positions that will allow you to heal yourself each and every day. Reiki healing, accompanied by your strong commitment to change and to advance yourself toward a better life, will heal you.

Healing Another Person

You do not really need to be deeply acquainted with another person to give them Reiki healing. You do not really need to know about his or her attitudes and the beliefs that guide them in life. You also do not need to make extra preparations in a person's attitudes and beliefs for them to receive Reiki healing from you. But all these things that I have just mentioned can make a big difference when you are healing someone else. When you are able to show that other person your love and compassion, you will be able to better help them get better. And when that person has real desire to be healed, you will also be able to better help them, merely by giving them your Reiki healing without asking anything for return.

As mentioned in the previous chapter, you can begin to give Reiki healing to people who are close to you, like your loved ones and your friends. You should be aware that when you do so, your deed of compassion will help them while improving your relationships with them. But you should be ready to go into a somewhat different mode when you begin use Reiki healing on other people. You will have to set aside your personal feelings for them that naturally arise because of your relationship.

You will begin the healing process by creating a suitable atmosphere in a sacred space. Make sure that you thoroughly wash your hands prior to and after completing the healing process. It is ideal that you enlighten the person that you will heal on the process and that you are about to perform and make them feel comfortable. Appease any apprehensions that they may have by telling them the Reiki energies are an intelligent energy. They will not receive more than they should. Ask for their consent to lay both your hands on them and ensure that you do not inappropriately interfere upon their own personal space. You can ask the recipient to either lie down on a bed or sit in a chair. Just make sure that they will feel comfortable when they begin drifting off to sleep during the healing process.

How to Adopt a Healing Attitude

Prior to beginning a Reiki healing session, you need to make an affirmation to yourself that after the healing process is over, you or the person you are healing will have more health and happiness. You need to prepare yourself by letting go of the things from your past that have given you pain and misery so you can fully accept a new future that is brighter and happier. If you are healing another person, ask them to prepare themselves in seeing things in a different manner and that they should be willing to release all their hurts and aches.

Invoke peaceful emotions to come to you and know that no other emotion is required in your healing process, except love. Allow yourself to sense an absolute love for yourself, for the other person that you wish to heal. Allow yourself to feel that you have complete trust and good intentions for the well-being of the person you want to heal and that your desire is to alleviate him or her from all the pains and suffering they are going through. You also need to make an affirmation that other people's issues and problems are not necessarily your problem and you do not need or want them in your life.

Know and feel in your heart that you do not mean to take another person's problem. Instead, you trust that, through divine healing, their pains and sufferings will be neutralized and that the darkness they have deep within will be changed into light. Finally, you need to make an affirmation of your intention to perform a Reiki healing and that you feel your connection with the source of Reiki energy is continuously strengthened. You need to believe that the Reiki healing that you are about to give is for the greatest good. Have faith that you will be guided and that the healing process has already started.

How to Create a Sacred Space

It is ideal for you to set up an atmosphere that is free from a lot of interruptions from other sources of energy when you are completing the Reiki healing process, especially when you are healing another person. Make sure that you will not be interrupted when you are doing the healing procedures. Make your surroundings as tranquil and as comfortable as you can. Turn off your cellular phone and if possible, place a "Do not disturb" signage on the door. The objective is for you to have a sacred space where you will not be disturbed.

You easily create a sacred space by reciting a prayer to God and to the angels. Ask them to sanctify the healing space you will use with their unconditional love. Request that they remove any unwanted energies from the area. When you ask God and the angels to sanctify your space, imagine in your head that the act is already being done. Know that your intention alone is powerful enough. Visualize a big golden bubble around the space that you want to be cleansed and protected. When you are able to do so, that can definitely become a sacred space.

It is also helpful if you can burn fragrance sticks and candles. You can play a gentle and soothing music to help establish a calm atmosphere in your healing area. It can also greatly help your recipient or the person you are healing to feel calm and relaxed during the process. When you have completed the healing process, it is ideal to give gratitude for the sacred area you have been endowed. Slowly visualize the golden bubble vanishing from the area.

Get Help

Before you begin your Reiki healing session, ask guidance and pray to God. You can also seek guidance from your Reiki Masters and Teachers in spirit and request them to bless and guide you when you are healing yourself or another person. Ask them to bestow their love to heal whoever you intend to receive your healing. Pray to God that His unconditional love will take away all the pains and sufferings you feel. Ask Him to guide you toward happiness. Believe in your heart that the Reiki healing system acts for the greater good at all times. Have faith that no matter what will happen during and after the healing process, know that is the right thing and the best for you. After you have completed your Reiki healing session, give gratitude to all who have given help and guidance to you.

Protection

There are some Reiki healers and spiritual people who feel that they require protection when performing Reiki healing. But many Reiki Masters believe that when you feel that you need protection, it can essentially indicate a reflex that is based on fear. When you continuously seek and use protection when healing, you are actually confirming your own weakness and helplessness. Do you believe that you need protection when you are walking down the street? Many people rely in their common sense in staying away from bad people, things and places. When you invoke your sacred space where you will hold your healing session, and when you say your prayer for guidance, you will acquire the protection you require. You just need to have faith.

Help Reiki Energy to Flow

You need to believe that you are actually a divine being because you are a part of God. You need to believe that when you have become attuned with Reiki energies, you have also become a channel for divine love. Before you begin your Reiki healing session, invoke a feeling in your heart that a chakra is spinning around and around inside you and you have unconditional love for all things flowing from within you. Visualize a wonderful beam of healing light coming from above your head straight to your head and downward toward your various chakras and, finally, into your heart chakra.

Visualize the light moving from your heart chakra down toward each of your arms into the palm of each of your hands. And then imagine a ray of light coming out from the palms of your recipient. Imagine those lights going directly into the back of your hands, which further enhance the rays of light already stretching out of your palms. Have faith that because your great love and because the unconditional love of all the Divine healers, all your pains and sufferings will be truly healed.

Have faith that true healing will occur. No matter what you do, the outcome will always be for your best welfare. But you should also be aware that the healing that you will receive will be intensified by the power of your intention to heal, by the power of the unconditional love and compassion you feel and by the prayers for healing you recite.

How to Place Your Hands During Healing

When you are Reiki 1 level, it is always ideal to actually position your hand on the body of the person you are healing. But you need to make sure that you always do this with utmost respect for the body and personal space of the person you intend to heal. Make it a habit to ask your client prior to the actual healing session and several times during the session if he or she feels comfortable when you place your hands on specific positions. You should always be mindful of what is and is not acceptable for your recipient.

Ask your recipients explicitly about their feelings for each hand placement. Make sure that you always employ discretion. It may seem appropriate to put your hand on the chest of a man but it is not acceptable to do the same with a woman. On the same note, you should be aware that the base chakra is one place that frequently requires a lot of healing but you are not supposed to place your hand on it. The best way for you to get through any discomfort or embarrassment is to explicitly ask the person you want to heal if he or she agrees with what you are about to do. Do this before you even start the healing session so the session can flow more naturally.

The set of hand positions recommended by Dr. Usui for Reiki healing are normally placed over the various chakras. A lot of the hand positions are placed around the head because it is one of the areas with great significance. You need to be mindful of where you place your hands and how long you keep them in a specific position. You should always keep in mind that the Reiki energies naturally flow to the location where it is most required. Therefore, it is always better to keep your hands on certain positions that are most comfortable for you while making the most contact with your two hands.

If your healing session is for less than an hour, it is ideal to spend a minimum of 10 minutes on the head. Just follow your own intuition and the divine guidance to discern where you are supposed to put your hands. If you or your recipient is complaining of a bad knee, you may sense that you need to spend more time placing your hands on that hurting knee. When you feel guided to go back to your or your recipient's heart chakra because you sense it requires more healing, feel free to do so.

Everything is Connected

You should be aware that everything in the universe is linked to one another. Everything, no matter how great or insignificant, consists of the same fundamental energy. We all came from just one source. The senses of our crown chakras allow us to know that all of us are part of just one universal consciousness and all things are one. This feeling is referred to as "Divine Love" – an awareness of the harmony of all things. In spite of the feelings of individualism we may have, we will sense that harmony and that oneness of all things, whether living or non-living, in all planes of consciousness. You need to be aware that this is such a great and powerful thing and that this oneness is far greater than the union of all group consciousness of men.

It is far greater than the union of all consciousness that revolves around our own sun because it powerfully connects the countless billions of galaxies existing in the universe and all the things that exist within. This oneness signifies that all of us are eternally in contact with all other things, no matter where those things may be. As a Reiki healer, you can make use of this connection to convey Reiki energies to absolutely anything. Use this connection to convey the healing powers of Reiki toward yourself or to another person you wish to heal.

Chapter 11: History Of Reiki

Reiki actually has a bit of a controversial history, and few realise that Reiki was once in danger of becoming an extinct art form. The United States had control of Japan in the years following World War II, and prohibited the use of any medical practices besides those approved by Western standards. Japanese groups who were fond of Reiki formed a secret society so they could continue their Reiki practice. They only practiced among their group and did not talk about Reiki to any outsiders, for fear of being caught. This nearly caused a complete halt of all exposure, learning and therefore spreading of Reiki. Japanese residents who were inclined to learn about it were forced to travel to the United States to learn a Westernised version of the practice. That is why most Reiki practiced today is a combination of the traditional Japanese Reiki and Western varieties. It also helps to explain why there are so many versions of Reiki history. Below are the histories of Japanese and Western Reiki, and some great insight as to how the two intertwine.

Mikao Usui: The Founder of Japanese Reiki

Mikao Usui was better known as Usui Sensei by his pupils. He was born on August 15, 1865 near what is now Nagoya in present day Japan. It is theorised that he joined a Buddhist school when he was four. He studied kiko, which is a subject on healing and health through the development and usage of life energy. These treatments required the practitioner to establish and increase, and then simply deplete his own sacred life energy while performing treatments. This was a source of major concern for Usui, and he tried to formulate a way to heal without depleting his own energy.

Usui loved learning and studied hard while at school. He also travelled overseas to China and Europe to continue his education, studying psychology, religion, medicine including divination, a popular subject for Asian students.

During one Buddhist meditation session, Usui felt a great energy entering his chakras, which gave him an expansive spiritual light and an understanding of how to resolve personal problems. Some legends assert that he found the energy when he stubbed his toe while running down a hill after meditating. He allegedly rubbed his foot after the fall, and a great energy transferred into his foot, healing the pain immediately. Usui was so excited about the energy that he directly went to share the power with his family. He practiced his newfound ability on them, further developing his skills as a healer by using a combination of his spiritual knowledge, philosophy studies and religious disciplines. He called it the Shin-Shin Kai-Zen Usui Reiki Ryo-Ho, or just Reiki for short, as it is now more widely known.

Usui became more and more skilled at his Reiki healing the more he practiced. He eventually wanted to share the practice with others so he could help more people, and opened a public practice in Tokyo in 1922. Here he not only had the chance to heal others, but teach Reiki to students who were also interested in becoming Reiki healers. Word about the Reiki centre got out, and soon people were coming from afar and waiting in long lines just to receive the services they craved.

In 1923, Tokyo suffered from an earthquake, which started a citywide fire. There were severely injured victims who sought Usui's practice for relief from their pain and cures to their mental and physical problems. The centre soon became too small for the extreme demand Usui was generating for his excellent practice, and he had to open a bigger place for his patients. He built a house right outside of Tokyo and transferred the practice there in 1925. He also started travelling the country to treat patients who requested house visits. Unfortunately, during one of his travels to Fukuyama, he caught an illness and abruptly died. He was sixty-two years old when he passed away.

Usui helped many people throughout his lifetime by healing problems of both the mind and body. He also taught many other teachers, who helped to pass down this Japanese tradition to generation after generation.

Although this is the accurate history of traditional Reiki, there are many other stories circulated when it comes to Western Reiki. There was one major player that shaped the history of Western Reiki, and her story follows.

The Origins of Western Reiki: Mrs. Takata

On Christmas Eve of 1900, a girl named Hawayo was born in Kauai, Hawaii to Japanese immigrant parents. Her father worked for a sugar cane plantation, and eventually Hawayo worked at the same place, and ended up marrying the bookkeeper of the plantation. Saichi Takata and Hawayo had two children together, but unfortunately, Saichi died in 1930 at 34 years old, and the widowed Mrs. Takata was forced to raise the children on her own.

Mrs. Takata worked hard to provide for her family, and the stress that came with it eventually took a toll on her health. She developed a serious lung condition, experienced severe abdominal pain and also suffered from a nervous breakdown. During this troubling time, her sister passed away, and Mrs. Takata had to travel back to Japan, where her parents had relocated, to let them know the news.

While she was there, she decided to seek help with her own medical condition. The Doctors in Japan informed her that she was suffering from a tumour, asthma, appendicitis and gallstones. While she was told to prepare for surgery, she instead chose to see a man named Hayashi Sensei who owned a Reiki clinic to learn more about his practice.

Although unfamiliar with Reiki, Mrs. Takata was intrigued because the Reiki practitioners diagnosed her with the same conditions the hospital had. She decided that exploring the option of Reiki treatments may be worth seeking, and started out with two treatments per day. The heat coming from the practitioners' hands was so hot that she suspected they were tricking her by using some sort of secret equipment to help them. One day, she grabbed the long sleeve of a kimono worn by a practitioner, expecting to find the secret to the mysterious heat, but was surprised to find nothing dubious at all. Bewildered, she explained to the startled practitioner what she was looking for, and he simply laughed, then explained to her how Reiki worked.

Mrs. Takata kept getting better, and was entirely healed of her afflictions within four months. She was so impressed that she decided to learn the art herself. She became a First Degree Reiki practitioner in 1936, worked for Dr. Hayashi for one year, and then received her Second Degree Reiki. Mrs. Takata went back to Hawaii in 1937, and Hayashi Sensei met her there with his daughter, and fulfilled their plans to bring Reiki to Hawaii. In 1938, Sensei established Takata as a Reiki Master.

Takata established several Reiki centres in Hawaii, giving treatments as well as teaching students up to the Second Degree Reiki. She taught Reiki to her patients' family members, and they were encouraged to practice Reiki at home for the patient. Takata strayed from traditional Reiki by simplifying the hand motions into eight standardized movements. This made Reiki easier to learn for beginners. She also began charging $10,000 for a Reiki degree, a training session that took only a weekend to complete. This was in contrast to traditional Reiki, which charged nothing or only a nominal fee to learn Reiki. Although some saw this as Takata turning her Reiki teachings into a selfish attempt to take others' money, others thought she was merely trying to establish respect for the degrees. Charging such a large amount made the degrees much more exclusive, and only affordable to those who took Reiki very seriously and willing to spend the $10,000 on a degree.

Takata continued to practice and teach others Reiki until she passed away in 1980. She was the first to bring Reiki into the western world, and was the cause of Reiki gaining so much popularity, as well. Before her death, Takata taught 22 Reiki Masters, who all began teaching others.

Although Usui and Takata may have had different ideas when it comes to applying and teaching Reiki to others, both should be acknowledged for their active roles in establishing and spreading the popularity of Reiki.

Chapter 12: How To Become A Reiki Master

The right way for how to turn into a Reiki expert can depend to an extensive degree on your inspirations. What is your arrangement once you have attained to the objective? Would you like to set up a Reiki hone? Would you like to utilize Reiki for recuperating? Would you like to thus instruct others? Then again would you say you are most inspired by the individual advantages, for example, enhanced self-acknowledgment?

It just bodes well that different methods for how to turn into a Reiki expert may be suitable relying upon how you plan to utilize and apply this superb device for vitality recuperating and self-acknowledgment!

In fact, numerous individuals ignore the self-acknowledgment advantages of Reiki. While numerous perceive that it is connected with vitality mending, the conceivable outcomes for internal equalization and mindfulness ought not be reduced.

Choices For How To Become A Reiki Master

The best place to begin is to pose a couple of straight forward inquiries:

Improve in a classroom situation?

Will you need reported affirmation?

Do you as of now have the business aptitudes to work a business?

Does your advantage lie in recuperating or in self-acknowledgment?

After that, you can assess the different methodologies and locate the particular case that best matches your own inclinations, your learning style, and your goals!

Generally, individuals got preparing in Reiki by adjusting to a Reiki expert. There was a methodology of working through the three levels of Reiki, with attunements occurring at every stage. These attunements to Reiki must be performed under the direction of the expert, and just an expert is qualified to perform them. Numerous experts contrived long courses for every level. These are a bit much, but rather from a business point of view they appeared well and good. Surely, by means of this methodology turning into a Reiki maser can cost near to $10,000. What's more, it can take a couple of years!

Those time gauges and expense appraisals speak to the great. There are likewise weekend workshops which you can go to, basically finishing a lever every weekend, so you can be qualified and guaranteed in three weekends.

None of this sets you up for running a practice from an organization or business viewpoint. However, it does get you qualified as a Reiki expert. You can then independently add to the business aptitudes required for achievement! There are additionally online techniques for how to turn into a Reiki expert. Despite the fact that these were at first scowled upon by conventional bosses, without a doubt the great ones were produced by extremely experienced experts who needed to have the capacity to achieve a more extensive group of onlookers. You see there are two schools of thought among the Reiki tip top. Some accept that it ought to be elite and hard controlled. Others need to spread the craftsmanship to however many individuals as could be allowed.

One of the huge advantages of the online Reiki courses is that you get the chance to finish them at your own pace. The other real playing point is that they are substantially less costly than the more customary methodologies.

At long last, some of them join business and organization preparing too, so you are exhaustively arranged for running your practice.

In case you're perusing this you presumably have some level enthusiasm for finding out about reiki or perhaps figuring out how to turn into a reiki expert.

Chapter 13: The Five Phases Of The Chi Cycle

Matter, with all its condensed Chi, being governed by the Cosmic Chi and being this influence directed by the Celestial Chi, nourishing itself with the Telluric Chi results in life. These influences and transformations are given within a polar Universe (positive-negative) manifested by the separation of Yin and Yang.

In this universe, everything will manifest within a constant oscillation between Yin and Yang. The different states through which Chi travels from Yin to Yang and vice versa, as well as the laws that this transit follows have been described by the Taoists in the Five Phases of the Chi Cycle.

Chi adopts certain characteristics during its passage through each of the phases. These phases are symbolically named by the elements of nature in which these characteristics are evidently reflected. The Five Phases are called the Phase of Fire, Earth, Metal, Water, and Wood. These are the characteristics that Chi adopts at each stage of its Yin-Yang transit.

The Five Phases of the Chi Cycle describe the dynamics of every cyclic movement in the universe, and as we have already seen in defining the concepts of Yin and Yang, the entire universe is a cyclic alternation, so everything is subject to the laws described in The Five Phases.

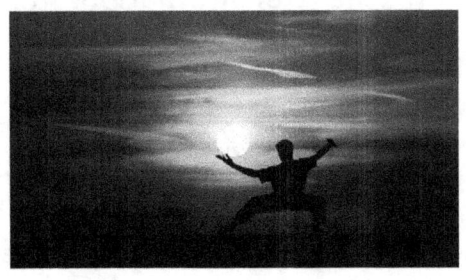

This continuous cycle is repeated in every being and every manifestation of the universe because everything is subject to Yin-Yang duality and nothing remains static. The formation and destruction of the stars and the life cycle of each being, the different biological processes that occur inside living beings. Everything is subject to this cycle.

•In the Fire phase, Chi is hot and rising, reaching the maximum expression of Yang. It is the energy that surpasses matter and expands abroad. It is the heat, the immaterial, the explosion, the culmination, the transformation. It's the summer, the plethora, the noon, the youth.

•In the Earth phase, Chi is more passive, temperate and binder. The Earth phase welcomes free energy and inert matter and unites them to form new manifestations of Chi. It is the center of the Chi Cycle, to which it returns after each phase and from which it leaves to the next cycle. It is the form, the result, the fruit and also the raw material for the new cycle. Agglutinate, amalgam, digest, equate. It is the harvest season, halftime, maturity, the beginning of the afternoon.

• In the Metal phase, Chi is contractive, delimiter, differentiator, selective. The Yang that was tempered in the Earth Phase now begins to descend towards its Yin aspect. The Chi of Metal tends to condense and collect, infusing the matter of energy, The Chi of Metal encourages the matter of energy, fills it with the Chi of life and puts pressure from the inside to keep outside the outside. It is condensation, internalization. It is the autumn, the entrance in the high ages, the late afternoon.

• In the Water phase, Chi descends and becomes paralyzed, reaching the maximum expression of the Yin, it is the materialization. The movement and the change come here to their minimum expression. Energy has been imbued in the matter and is now endowed with a stable structure. The validity for the structure is selected and that superfluous is discarded and discarded. Chi is preserved imbued in matter. It is the reign of immobility. The dance is frozen, but Chi continues its path of transformation: the modifying potential of Yang is stored in the matter and will be released under the right circumstance. The Yin awaits the time to return the energy received. It is the seed, wait for it. It is winter and cold, old age, night.

•In the Wood phase, Chi expands and mobilizes. Wood Chi is the energy that governs matter. "Yin retains Yang. Yang rules the Yin", as the maxim says. The Chi retained in the matter is claimed, influenced, mobilized from the outside, and dragging the matter behind it, the endowment of mobility and the movement begins to adapt to new circumstances, expansion and life again. It is the Yang giving life to the Yin, heating it. It is movement, growth and expansion, adaptation. It is spring, childhood, and morning.

Each being, animate or inanimate, that manifests itself in nature is constituted by a multitude of different chis, of a more yin or more yang nature and that respond to one or another phase of the Chi Cycle. All these influences endow the being in the question of its own characteristics, and the harmony between all these forces allows that being to last for a certain time. The imbalance of all these influences that constitute the being derives in the degradation of the misno or its evolution to a new state because everything in nature tends to look for a point of balance.

The balance between yin, yang and the chi corresponding to the different phases of the Chi Cycle, in addition to others closer to the Western mentality such as the liquid-heat and matter-energy ratio, are the basis for the understanding of health and disease from the perspective of Chinese culture.

We already know that the chi that is in each of the phases will have certain determined characteristics, but the different chi does not exist in isolation but interact with the chi of the other cycles accompanying the constant movement. The influences exerted between chi of different nature are studied under two different natures: the food or growth cycle and the control cycle.

In the Growth Cycle the Chi of each phase feeds or powers that of the next phase. This is traditionally expressed as "the mother feeds the child": the Water Phase feeds the Wood Phase, the Fire Phase, etc.

On the other hand, in the Control Cycle, we usually say that "the counselor moderates the emperor": the Chi of the Water Phase controls that of the Fire Phase, this one of metal, etc.

The beings and manifestations of this universe will show the preponderance of some of these forms of manifestation of Chi. The relationships between the different natures of Chi will help us to understand the relationships between different beings and the relationships that are established between the internal vital processes of each living being.

Consider the following example: The new president of a company, about forty years old (land) that displaces and imposes its criteria against those previously maintained by the former President, now an elder (water) using to reach his goals energy of young employees (fire). Thus, fire feeds the earth that in turn controls the water. But if the former president felt that his successor abused his position, he could establish his authority directly over the employees. So water would control the fire, restoring balance by restricting support for the land.

The Macrocosm and the Microcosm

In the outer universe (macrocosm), Yin and Yang are manifested in the main climatic periods of summer and winter. The passage from one to another is carried out through different stations that correspond to the Five Phases of Energy: Winter (maximum Yin, predominance of Water Chi), Spring (predominance of Wood Chi), Summer (Fire Chi), Late summer, harvest and intermediate seasons (Earth Chi), Autumn (Metal Chi) and we start again.

Another macrocosmic cycle of Yin and Yang interaction is the day-night cycle. Here, in the same way, the Chi passes from its manifestation plus Yin to the most Yang and again to the Yin through the five specified phases: The Fire Chi corresponds to noon (solar time), period of maximum Yang; at midnight we will find the predominance of the Water Chi, the Wood Chi will correspond to the morning, the first hours of the afternoon will bring the Earth Chi and the last hours before the night will impose the Metal Chi.

An obvious macrocosmic cycle would be that of the tides, governed by the direct influences of the Sun and the Moon, which in turn follow their own cycles. The human being, within nature, follows his own Chi cycle, while participating in the dance of the universe by being influenced by the cycles that surround him and in turn intervening with his own cycle, especially as a global Human Being. There are other macrocosmic cycles, but their influence is less evident than that of these main cycles because it is exerted by more subtle energies that, as we have already mentioned, lack the capacity to exert immediate apparent changes on the material planes.

For its part, the organism of living beings maintains its own internal cycles of Yin-Yang alternation: sleep and wakefulness may be the most obvious cycle, but there is also activity-rest, food-fasting, inspiration-expiration, systole-diastole, contraction-strain, etc. These cycles of the internal universe (microcosmic) follow the same laws as the macrocosmic cycles and in them, the Chi also adopts the characteristics of each of the Five Phases of the Chi Cycle.

The internal cycles of living beings (microcosms) are connected with the cycles of the rest of the Universe (external, macrocosmic) because otherwise, living beings could not access the Cosmic Chi and the Celestial Chi, without which life is not possible.

Thus, with the rising of the Sun, the expansive Chi of the Wood seizes us, which activates us throughout the morning. At noon, our body has to adapt to the moment of maximum energy under the influence of Fire Chi. Moments later we have entered the moment of maximum apogee of the monotonous Chi of the Earth, and throughout the afternoon we feel it's slow and reflective energy. When the Sun already falls and the Chi of the Metal preponderates, our body begins to internalize its energy preparing for the night, during which the Chi of the Water adds us to the stillness. We receive these same influences during the annual cycle of the seasons.

The internal and external cycles complement and compensate in complex interactions, sometimes obvious and sometimes difficult to perceive.

The Human Being receives its most direct influences from the Sun and the Earth (Telluric Chi and Cosmic Chi respectively), our main sources of Chi. The breakage of our synchronism with these external sources of Chi has consequences that cannot be expected: when the demands of civilization break the natural rhythm of sleep-wakefulness or activity-rest, they interfere with the mechanism of our body to absorb the different qualities of Chi. The vitality of our body decreases and our mind loses clarity. Our biological mechanism stops adjusting and begins to deteriorate more rapidly. The disease will find the door open and can begin to develop within us.

In the common person, the Cosmic Chi enters indirectly through breathing and feeding. Breathing incorporates into our body the Chi that is in our environment at all times and different foods store different concentrations of different types of Chi.

Inhabiting inadequate spaces makes us constantly receive low-quality Chi. The intake of a monotonous diet can cause us to receive too much or too little of any of the types of Chi. Thus, if we eat too many foods in which Chi plus Yang predominate, our body will present a Yang preponderance. The same will happen if we abuse Yin food in excess. On the other hand, the different organs and tissues of our body consume certain qualities of Chi to perform their tasks. If they do not have them, they tire and wear out prematurely.

Additionally, much of the Chi that we acquire is consumed in the activity of compensation for external influences and internal processes, so that the more unbalanced the different qualities of Chi are in our being, the more easily we will lose synchronicity with the medium and our own internal processes. Chi can also manifest itself in ways that are harmful to the human being: excessive heat, excessive humidity are the pathogenic clients of Chinese medicine. Keep our Chi at an optimal level that protects us from these harmful influences. They are also essential for the conservation of health and it is our internal Chi that has to prevent the entrance of these climates to the organism.

Chapter 14: Performing A Treatment

Client comfort will have a significant impact on your ability to deliver an effective treatment. Uncomfortable clients tend to close themselves off to treatments, resisting energy delivery.

If a client is coming to you, be sure to have a space prepared that is conducive to creating a relaxed and peaceful environment.

A massage table is perfect for delivering Reiki treatments. Playing soft meditative background music may prove helpful. Be careful with incense. Some clients will appreciate it, others may not. The temperature of the room should also be kept at a temperature that is not too cold or too warm, if possible.

When the client is lying on the table, it is often helpful to cover them with a light blanket. This will help them feel more secure in what could often prove a very emotionally intimate setting. Be sure to check comfort levels in terms of temperature before proceeding.

When the client is ready to start the treatment ask them to lie on their back on the table. For newer clients it will be especially helpful if you take a minute or two to just explain what you are doing.

Once ready, be sure to ask permission from the client to proceed with the treatment. Start with some meditative breathing exercises with the client to help them relax. Deep breath in and out a few times will do the trick.

One of the things you will have to decide as a practitioner is whether to touch the client as part of the treatment or whether to just use a beaming approach. There are good reasons for both, but for the most part I would suggest that unless your client is totally comfortable with touch, a beam approach may prove more comfortable for most clients.

There are some comfort touch points that generally will not cause discomfort for a client. These are to let the client know where you are, even when their eyes are closed.

These points are only useful if you only use a very light non invasive touch. Comfort touch points are generally only useful for newer clients. Use your better judgment as to whether the client will feel more or less comfortable if you use touch points.

Key treatment and comfort touch points

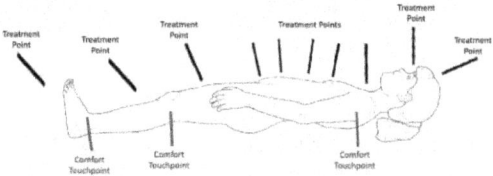

Treating the body, you will be moving around the body, starting at the crown, working your way down the body all the way to the soles of the feet. The direction you move is the same as for the vortex symbol, driven by which hemisphere you are in. (Clockwise in the southern hemisphere and anti-clockwise in the northern hemisphere) Spend a few minutes at each treatment point transmitting energy to your client. You will soon learn to sense whether more or less energy is required at a particular treatment point. Use your own judgment to decide when to move on.

When the top to bottom treatment is completed have the client turn face down and repeat the treatment pattern.

You will notice that from crown to root the treatment points are in line with traditionally known chakra centers of the body. Chakras connect energy points of the body together. Take advantage of this connectivity for delivery of your treatments by transmitting energy into the general vicinity of the chakra points.

In the second degree you will start learning how to sense problems with the client's energy structures. Since being a Reiki practitioner does not require that you have advanced knowledge of anatomy, it may be useful to use chakra points as reference points for recording your client treatment data.

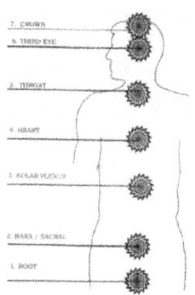

{chakra points}

Typical treatments can take anywhere between 30 - 60 minutes. There are no set rules for this. It is totally up to you and your sense of the client energy systems to treat for as long as is necessary. When you start feeling the client demand for energy reduce it is time to move on to the next treatment point.

If you are using a touch based treatment approach be aware that for most clients, throat, heart and root chakra treatment points will prove especially uncomfortable. To reduce the discomfort, there are some hand positions that will help you with this.

Throat : It is better not to wrap your hands around the client's throat, especially across the front of the throat. Rather place your hands, underneath the neck, palms facing up and inwards. Stand behind the client in the crown position facing towards the clients' body.

Heart Chakra : Position yourself next to the client. Pointing away from yourself create a "T" with your hands. Touch on the client's breastbone at the heart center position.

{Heart Chakra hand position}

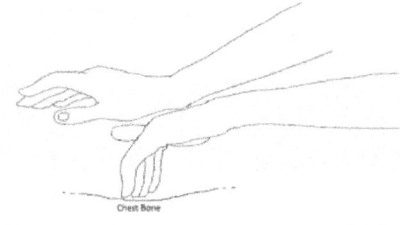

Root Chakra : Use similar hand positioning to the Heart Chakra, however place the bottom hand between the navel and root on the body. Remember to apply gentle touch. Angle the palms slightly in the direction of the root chakra.

If you opt to use the beaming approach, place yourself next to the body (crown from the top and feet from the bottom) and beam energy towards the client and the respective treatment points. Direct the palms of your hands towards the client.

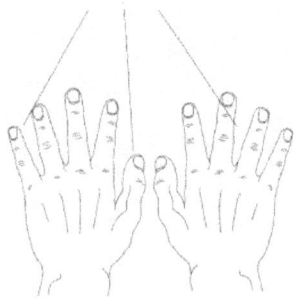

Follow the same treatment pattern as for the touch based approach.

If you have a limited amount of time to treat a client and you are aware of a localized issue you can focus your treatment on the affected areas only.

When the treatment is completed

Very often clients will experience a state of high emotion and even euphoria from a Reiki treatment.

When the treatment is completed be sure to give the client a little time to collect themselves before kicking them out of your treatment space.

If they have fallen asleep, do wake them up gently but be sure that they have a few minutes, so make sure not to cram clients in back to back.

One after treatment grounding technique is particularly useful to help clients re-establish their connection to reality. Help the client reinitialize their sense by instructing them to touch, feel and sense something. When they touch the object (could be the massage table or the blanket...) instruct them to focus on the temperature of the object, the texture of the object and generally how it feels. Instruct them to do so with another.

Protecting yourself from your clients

Because you are connecting with a client in a very fundamental way, working with their base energy systems, it becomes very easy for you to take on some of the client's energy. Even though you can focus the direction of energy flow towards the client, any energy connection that you establish will be a two way connection.

This is more true when your personal relationship grows beyond a simple practitioner / client relationship.

This energy "blowback" can affect you in very negative ways. It can even be carried between clients. It is very important that you protect yourself and take care of yourself properly.

If you continue your studies you may learn how to use the two way flow of energy to enhance your healing abilities. This will require further study that goes beyond the scope of the First Degree.

At all times remain disconnected from the outcome.

Although, as a practitioner, it will be useful for you to track the results of your treatments, it is very important to consider this in a clinical way. If you get emotionally attached to your success and failures, your fear of failure will cloud your success. You will also end up passing your anxiety through to your client.

Be confident that your treatment has achieved it's intended outcome, no matter what.

If you struggle with confidence, practice makes perfect. Practice, practice and then practice some more. Meditation is helpful for establishing a neutral balance in your mind.

Visualizeprotection.
Your thoughts are what drives your treatment. Visualize filtration or barriers preventing client energy from blowing back on you. This will reduce or eliminate completely the negative affects that could be passed back to you. Blue or white light is particularly cleansing and protective.

Visualize yourself completely engulfed with light. Visualize your treatment flow outwards through the light towards your client and the light neutralizing any energy that returns.

Practice doing this until it becomes like breathing. Automatic.

Ground yourself and your client. In every treatment there will be excess energy not needed or used by your client or yourself as part of this process. This energy needs to go somewhere.

The best way to get rid of excess energy is to create a visualized connection to the ground for both you and your client. Excess energy can be drained away from your client into the ground. Energy not passed through to your client, or used to replenish your own energy systems, will also be channeled out.

In addition to visualizations also take advantage of simple breathing exercises, which can be used to help your client prepare for receiving a treatment.

One exercise in particular is deep breath in

(4 count), hold (16 count), out 8 count. Repeat two or three times.

Have the client perform the preparatory exercises before every treatment. Use the Reiki Symbols diligently.

Using the symbols will significantly increase the focus of your treatment. This will strengthen directionality as well as the treatment.

The first degree symbol is particularly useful for this purpose. Cleans before and after treatments.

When treating someone there is always energy spillage which will attach to you. Energetic hygiene is important.

For your own personal health and to minimize transference between clients, take the time to clean your energy structures.

Start by simply washing your hands. Soap and water. Visualized light cleansing of your entire being is a very effective way to clean. Breathing exercises to help you focus your mind as part of your visualized cleansing will enhance this process.

Conclusion

Thank you again for downloading this book!

The next step is to apply all that you have learned from this book, and actively seek the improvement of yourself, the energizing of your chakras, and a better understanding of your environment, and how all things are connected.

Opening and recharging chakras takes time and practice. You must consistently do the techniques detailed in this book, and mind your thoughts, actions, words and interactions. Remember that everything, when reduced to its purest form, resonates with energy, and that you have the power to absorb or change that energy.

The seven chakras will help you stay in-tune with your body and mind. It will present you with opportunities to help your spirit grow in wisdom and strength. There are other minor chakras that you may also want to research about, and other methods that could help you recharge your chakras. Whichever method you choose, remember that you must never give up on this life changing, personal journey of discovery.

Thank you and good luck!

www.ingramcontent.com/pod-product-compliance
Lightning Source LLC
Chambersburg PA
CBHW072013070526
44583CB00015B/1457